Valvular Heart Disease
in Clinical Practice

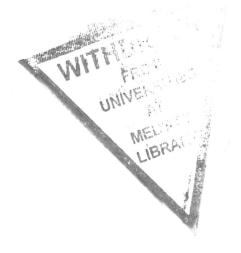

Michael Y. Henein
Editor

Valvular Heart Disease in Clinical Practice

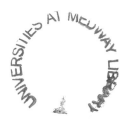

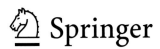 Springer

Editor
Michael Y. Henein
Consultant Cardiologist
Umea Heart Centre
Umea University
Sweden

ISBN: 978-1-84800-274-6   e-ISBN: 978-1-84800-275-3
DOI 10.1007/978-1-84800-275-3

British Library Cataloguing in Publication Data
A catalogue record for this book is available from the British Library

Library of Congress Control Number: 2008940632

Springer Science+Business Media
springer.com

Preface

Over the last three decades, major advances in the management of diseases of the valves have been seen. While cardiac catheterization was in the 1970s, the only means for confirming the diagnosis, Doppler echocardiography has become the corner stone for accurate assessment of valve disease, even in fetuses. Now not only the disease can be identified but also the rate of disease progression (e.g. leaflet calcification and stiffness) can be accurately measured and quantified by echocardiography and multislice/electron beam CT imaging. Surgical treatment of valve disease has also witnessed great advances, having moved from traditional valve replacement to sophisticated repair procedures and the use of extracorporeal pump support in some patients. Robotic valve surgery has also proved a great success, in well selected cases, and is expected to have a fruitful future. Furthermore, in special circumstances, conventional surgical valve excision has now been replaced by percutaneous catheter-based valve replacement for aortic and pulmonary disease. This approach reduces the risk from the surgery itself, avoids general anaesthesia and many potential post-operative complications.

This book discusses the practicalities of the diagnosis and treatment of the various aspects of common heart valve diseases, covering most clinical and surgical issues. It is designed to assist clinicians in the management of patients with valve disease and provide them with answers to many of the clinical questions that arise. With the rapid developments in medical technology, the management of valve diseases remains an exciting area for future research, the results of which should be incorporated in a future edition of this book.

I would like to take this opportunity to offer my sincere thanks to the other contributors to this book and also to our patients, without whom our knowledge on this and other cardiac diseases would have never matured.

Michael Y. Henein
London, UK
Umeà, Sweden

Contents

1 **The Mitral Valve Disease** 1
Michael Henein and John Pepper

2 **Aortic Valve Disease** 73
Michael Henein and Joseph Maalouf

3 **Right Heart Valve Disease** 155
Michael Henein

4 **Pulmonary Valve Disease** 195
Michael Henein and Wei Li

5 **Stress Echo in Valvular Heart Disease** 221
Eugenio Picano

6 **Valve Substitutes** 241
John Chambers

7 **Native and Prosthetic Valve Endocarditis** 265
Maurizio Galderisi and Sergio Mondillo

Index 289

Contributors

John Chambers, MD
Consultant Cardiologist
Head of Non-invasive Cardiology
St Thomas' Hospital,
London, UK

Maurizio Galderisim, MD
Director of Eclo-Lab,
Cardioangiology with CCU
Federico II University Hospital
Naples, Italy

Michael Henein, MD
Professor and Consultant Cardiologist
Umeà University Hospital
Heart Centre, Sweden

Wei Li, MD
Adult Congenital Heart Cardiologist
Royal Brompton Hospital
London, UK

Joseph Maalouf, MD
Professor of Medicine
Mayo Clinic
Rochester, Mennisota
USA

Sergio Mondillo, MD
Professor and Director of the Postgraduate School of
Cardiovascular Diseases of Cardiology
University of Siena
Siena, Italy

John Pepper, MD
Professor of Cardiothoracic Surgery
Imperial College London
Royal Brompton Hospital,
UK

Eugenio Picano, MD
Director
Institute of Clinical Physiology of Italian
National Research Council
Pisa, Italy

Michael Rigby, MD
Consultant Paediatric Cardiologist
Royal Brompton Hospital
London, UK

Mary Sheppard, MD
Consultant Pathologist
Royal Brompton Hospital
London, UK

Chapter 1
The Mitral Valve Disease

Michael Henein and John Pepper

Common causes of heart valve disease are rheumatic, calcific and less frequently congenital. With the significant decline in the incidence of rheumatic fever in Europe and North America over the last 50 years a parallel shift in the etiology of valve disease occurred with a fall in the incidence of rheumatic valve disease and an increase in the prevalence of degenerative valve pathology. Rheumatic valve disease, however, remains prevalent in the developing countries in Africa, South America and parts of Asia, particularly in areas with limited clinical services. The commonest valve involved with rheumatic pathology is the mitral valve, but this is not exclusive since aortic and tricuspid valves can also be involved [1]. The apparent contemporary increase in the diagnosis of valve disease results from the global increase in age of the population as well as the easy availability and routine use of echocardiography in cardiology clinics. Age affects the valves by making the leaflets thick with fibrous strands and adipose tissue deposition at the closure lines as well as increased calcium deposition. Isolated myxomatous changes may also occur in the valve fibrosa. This complex pathology eventually results in valve dysfunction. In an echocardiographic examination, such effects of age on valve leaflets should be carefully considered, particularly in patients with a suspected diagnosis of endocarditis since leaflet thickening may appear like small

M.Y. Henein (ed.), *Valvular Heart Disease in Clinical Practice*,
DOI 10.1007/978-1-84800-275-3_1,
© Springer-Verlag London Limited 2009

vegetations. They should also be distinguished from other small benign tumors, e.g., fibroelastoma.

Medical treatment of mild valve disease is limited, focusing mostly on prophylaxis against endocarditis. In more significant valve disease, medical treatment aims at optimizing the hemodynamics and consequently protecting against ventricular dysfunction. Surgical correction of valve disorder is the main conventional treatment of severe valve disease, particularly in patients with maintained ventricular function. Those with additional irreversible ventricular dysfunction may face significant surgical risk, thus medical therapy might be the best management option for them. In general, valve-related mortality is more prevalent in aortic valve disease than mitral valve disease, largely due to either sudden death from arrhythmia or the frequent development of left ventricular dysfunction that causes congestive heart failure. Other causes of death in valve disease are additional pathologies, e.g. coronary artery disease, endocarditis or arrhythmia. Overall valve surgery is 5–10 times less frequently performed than that for coronary artery disease [1].

Normal Mitral Valve Anatomy and Function

Optimum function of the mitral valve depends on the integral function of all its components: leaflets, chordae, annulus and papillary muscles in addition to the left atrium and the left ventricle. A normal mitral valve does not close passively. In addition to the pressure difference between the ventricle and the atrium in systole, the annular contraction and papillary muscle contraction play an important role in the competence of the mitral valve. The anterior mitral valve leaflet represents a continuation of the posterior aortic root wall. The D-shaped annular fibrous ring is located mainly posteriorly, although significant variability exists in different individuals. The normal diameter of the mitral annulus is approximately 3 cm with a circumference of 8–9 cm. The annulus is not a passive structure, so in addition to its normal movement towards the apex in systole, the contraction of the posterior myocardial muscle shortens its diameter by 25%, making annular dynamics a very important component in the mechanism of mitral valve competence. Left atrial cavity enlargement and shape change result in mitral annular dilatation and hence overall valve dysfunction and incompetence. With progressive increase in left atrial size and development of atrial fibrillation, the lost mechanical atrial activity significantly contributes to mitral valve incompetence and the development of mitral regurgitation. Likewise, atrial fibrillation itself has been shown to contribute to the enlargement of the left atrium and consequently, the development of mitral regurgitation. The two leaflets of the mitral valve meet at the medial and lateral commissures. The U-shaped anterior leaflet area is larger than the posterior leaflet by approximately 3–4 cm^2. The posterior leaflet is, however, wider and shorter than the anterior leaflet by approximately 1.5 cm^2. The posterior leaflet is made up of a number of scallops, commonly three. The two leaflets coapt at the zone of apposition leaving an overlapping segment 5 mm long. The chordal anatomy of the mitral valve is complicated, with around 12 primary chordae rising from each papillary muscle, which divide into secondaries and numerous tertiary branches which attach themselves to the margins of the two leaflets. In addition, a number of basal chordae also attach themselves to the ventricular surface of the two leaflets and to the commissures. The location of the chordae follows that of the papillary muscles antero-laterally and postero-medially. Any rupture or redundancy of the chordae or extra tissue in the leaflets results in mitral regurgitation.

The normal mitral valve orifice cross-sectional area is approximately 5.0 cm^2, Figure 1.1 allowing left ventricular filling to occur predominantly in early diastole (approximately two-thirds of stoke volume) at a peak rate of 500–1000 ml/s (Figure 2.1). The remaining one-third of the stroke volume passes through the mitral valve during atrial systole. During diastasis, ventricular volume remains unchanged [2]. With

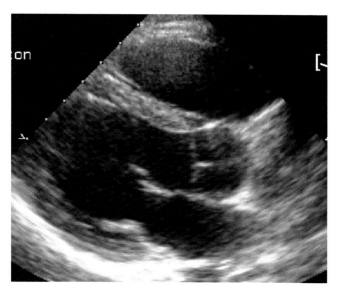

FIGURE 1.1.   Parasternal 2D long axis view showing anterior (extending from the posterior aortic wall) and posterior (extending from the left atrial posterior wall) mitral valve leaflets.

exercise and increase in heart rate, diastasis shortens and the early and late filling components approximate until they summate and become indistinguishable [3]. With age, the filling pattern reverses so that dominant left ventricular filling occurs in late diastole [4] Figure 1.2.

Mitral Stenosis

Congenital mitral stenosis: It is a relatively rare group of anomalies with considerable variations in the morphological features. Normally included in this diagnosis are cortriatriatum and supra-valvar mitral membrane, which can be identified from the four-chamber and long axis cross-sectional images Figure 1.3. Characteristically, color flow Doppler

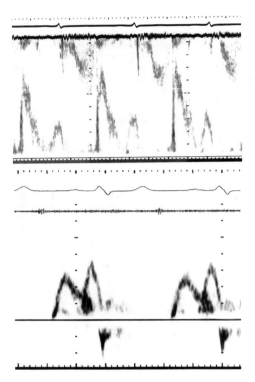

FIGURE 1.2. Transmitral Doppler flow velocities from a young subject showing dominant early diastolic component (*top*) and an elderly showing dominant late diastolic component (*bottom*).

reveals acceleration proximal to the mitral valve leaflets. It is not unusual, however, for the supra-valvar mitral stenosis to be associated with thickened mitral valve leaflets and chordal abnormalities. It is unusual to find isolated mitral valve stenosis. In addition to thickened and dysplastic leaflets, anomalies of the chordae and the papillary muscles may be seen. In the classical parachute mitral valve, all the chords insert into a single papillary muscle.

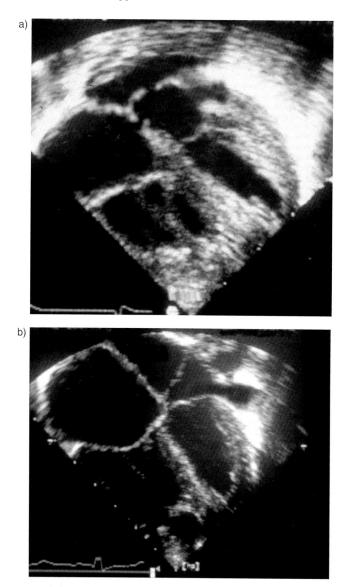

FIGURE 1.3. (**a,b**) Subcostal views from two patients with cortriatriatum, one parallel to mitral valve leaflets and the other at oblique angle. (**c**) Subcostal view from a patient with supra-valvar membrane.

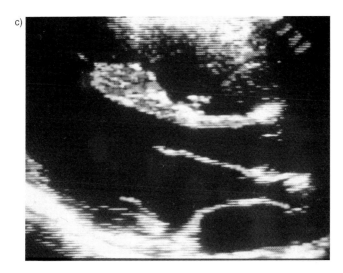

FIGURE 1.3. Continued

Rheumatic Mitral Stenosis

Pathophysiology: The most common cause of mitral stenosis is rheumatic valve disease. Rheumatic mitral stenosis affects 10/100,000, mainly in Asia, Africa and South America. The rheumatic process not only involves the leaflets but may also affect the chordae and the annulus causing fibrosis and super-imposed calcification. The rheumatic leaflets become thickened, fibrosed and the commissures fuse. The end result of this pathology is a fall in mitral valve area. Figure 1.4 the rigid movement of the leaflets and the commissural fusion together contribute to the limited blood flow across the mitral valve orifice and hence stenosis. It is not uncommon for the fibrotic process to involve the subvalvar apparatus in an aggressive way thus causing the flow-limiting level at the subvalvar region. In this case, the chordae are short and the inflow tract of the left ventricle becomes tunnel-like Figure 1.4. The important consequence of mitral stenosis is its effect on left atrial pressure, size and the pulmonary vasculature. As the

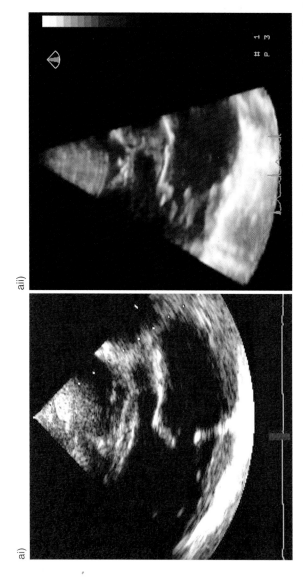

ai)   aii)

FIGURE 1.4. (**ai,aii**) Two-dimensional and 3D parasternal long axis view showing rheumatic mitral valve leaflets. Note the thickening and bowing of the anterior leaflet in diastole. (**b**) Similar view from a patient with fibrosed subvalvar apparatus causing subvalvar stenosis. (**c**) Mitral valve M-mode echogram from the same patient showing characteristic pattern of stiff rheumatic anterior leaflet in diastole and the anterior movement of the posterior leaflet.

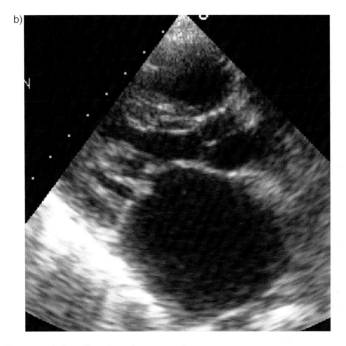

FIGURE 1.4.B Continued.

valve area falls further, left atrial emptying reduces, left atrial size and pressure increase and the pulmonary venous pressure also increases. Long-standing conditions may result in irreversible pulmonary hypertension secondary to the raised left atrial pressure. In most patients with rheumatic mitral valve disease, the left ventricle is normal in size and systolic function, unless the valve stenosis is severe and making the ventricle underfilled. With a valve area of 2.5 cm^2, symptoms start to appear as transmitral pressure drop becomes influenced by valve area, rhythm, duration of diastasis and ventricular diastolic function. With a valve area of less than 2.5 cm^2, peak left ventricular filling rate falls and diastasis is lost. This is of no physiological consequence at rest but with exercise left ventricular filling is only maintained by a significant rise in left atrial pressure and the pressure drop between the left atrium and left ventricle. As the valve area becomes progressively smaller, a pressure drop develops at rest. This is usually associated with a fall in cardiac output and increase in pulmonary vascular resistance. In severe mitral stenosis, the pressure difference between the left atrium and left ventricle may be as high as 25–30 mmHg. With severe mitral stenosis, valve area may become less than 1 cm^2 in comparison to the normal valve area of 5 cm^2. The increase in heart rate does not significantly change the effective mitral orifice area compared to the aortic stenotic area. This could be explained by the lesser number of commissures that assist in the opening of the mitral valve compared to those of the aortic valve. With exercise, particularly in patients with atrial fibrillation, diastolic time shortens and the fixed mitral valve area causes increased left atrial pressure and pulmonary venous pressure. Mitral valve area can also be affected by extensive annular calcification, which is a common finding in the elderly. This pathology is frequently seen in long standing hypertensives and tends to affect mainly the annulus and the proximal part of the leaflets but does not result in any significant hemodynamic picture of mitral stenosis. Left atrial emptying velocities can be somewhat raised reflecting only modest increase in atrioventricular pressure drop.

Complications of Mitral Stenosis

Left Atrial Dilatation

Progressive reduction in mitral valve orifice area causes progressive increase in left atrial pressure and size, particularly in the young and middle-aged patients. Progressive increase in left atrial pressure causes pulmonary venous hypertension. Left atrial dilatation is associated with reduction in its mechanical function which slows down intra-atrial swirling blood circulation. With progressive disease and development of atrial fibrillation, the circulation in the atrium becomes very sluggish and echocardiography may demonstrate spontaneous echo-contrast, which is particularly seen on transesophageal images. Such patients are given anti-coagulants in order to avoid clot formation and to reduce the risk of cerebrovascular accidents. Left atrial thrombus formation is very common in patients with severe mitral stenosis, almost one-fifth of those undergoing surgery have left atrial thrombus and in one-third of them the thrombus is restricted to the atrial appendage [5]. Even in patients with sinus rhythm, left atrial thrombus may form in those with dilated left atrium and spontaneous contrast and hence the need for anti-coagulation.

Atrial Fibrillation

It is the most common complication of mitral stenosis and its prevalence increases with age [6], being in 70% of patients in the thirties and in 80% of those in the fifties. The presence of pulmonary hypertension raises the prevalence of atrial fibrillation, being in 60% of patients [7]. The Framingham study estimated a 20-fold increase in the risk of stroke in patients with atrial fibrillation and mitral stenosis compared to only 5-fold increase in those without mitral valve disease [8]. Although the loss of left atrial appendage mechanical function has been proposed as a possible mechanism behind blood stagnation and thrombus formation [9], it is by no means the sole cause of thrombus formation. The combination of left atrial enlargement and asynchronous function in atrial fibrillation is the most likely underlying cause of thrombus formation.

Pulmonary Hypertension

With the increase in left atrial pressure, the pulmonary venous pressure increases followed by raised pulmonary arterial pressure. Pulmonary artery pressure usually reflects the degree of increase in left atrial pressure in mitral stenosis. It is very rare for pulmonary hypertension to develop with left atrial pressure less than 20 mmHg in the setting of isolated mitral stenosis. Despite that, discrepancy between the two may suggest a raised pulmonary vascular resistance or a primary etiology for pulmonary hypertension. Long standing mitral stenosis and pulmonary hypertension may result in irreversibly raised pulmonary vascular resistance; even a successful valve surgery and correction of mitral stenosis may not guarantee a normal pressure drop across the pulmonary bed of approximately 10–15 mmHg. Such patients may remain limited by breathlessness despite having successful mitral valve surgery [10].

Right Heart Disease

With the development of pulmonary hypertension, the right ventricle becomes hypertrophied and its cavity dilates with time. As right ventricular myocardium becomes stiff, diastolic pressures raise and are reflected on right atrial pressure and eventually right atrial dilatation occurs. Patients with rheumatic mitral valve disease may have additional tricuspid valve involvement, in particular the annulus dilates and causes significant tricuspid regurgitation. Patients with severe tricuspid regurgitation may develop fluid retention which needs careful management in order to maintain optimum left-sided cardiac output and obtain tissue perfusion. Long-standing significant tricuspid regurgitation itself and raised right atrial pressure may cause further deterioration of right ventricular function and congestive heart failure. By that stage, the myocardial damage is usually irreversible despite any successful mitral valve surgery. Fluid retention secondary to tricuspid valve disease should be carefully managed, particularly in patients subjected to mitral valve surgery, who may require the two valves replaced in the same setting. Once irreversible right ventricular myocardial dysfunction occurs, tricuspid valve surgery adds no symptomatic or prognostic clinical value. In contrast, it significantly increases the surgical risk and peri-operative morbidity.

Left Ventricular Dysfunction

In most cases with mitral stenosis, the left ventricle is normal in size and systolic function is well maintained. However, in some patients diastolic function may be abnormal with raised end-diastolic pressure. This picture could be related to additional pathologies, e.g., hypertension, diabetes or coronary artery disease rather than primary rheumatic myocardial disease. The latter was suggested years ago but no convincing evidence has ever substantiated. Left ventricular cavity dilatation is only seen in the presence of additional coronary artery disease.

Clinical Presentation

Symptoms: Patients with mild mitral stenosis may remain asymptomatic for years. As the disease progresses and valve area falls, the early symptoms are exertional breathlessness and fatigue. Breathlessness worsens as the mitral valve area progressively falls. With severe mitral stenosis, breathlessness is accompanied by orthopnea and paroxysmal nocturnal dyspnea. With the development of pulmonary hypertension, breathlessness becomes intolerable, even at rest. Patients who develop right ventricular dysfunction and tricuspid regurgitation may present with fluid retention as well as recurrent chest infection. Atrial fibrillation may be the early symptom in patients with mitral stenosis, particularly causing palpitations on exercise. Major cerebrovascular accidents or transient ischemic attacks may be the presenting symptom in ignored cases. Mitral stenosis may be detected for the first time during pregnancy as patients complain of disproportionate breathlessness.

Physical examination: The characteristic auscultatory features of rheumatic mitral stenosis are an opening snap in early diastole, mid-diastolic murmur and loud first heart sound. The opening snap is caused by the abrupt tension that develops in the fibrosed anterior leaflet at the termination of the opening movement. The opening snap is best heard at the apex; it becomes closer to the second heart sound as left atrial pressure rises and mitral valve is forced to open early. The opening snap is usually absent when the leaflets become heavily calcified. The diastolic murmur is low pitched and maximal at the apex. It is caused by increased blood flow velocity between the left atrium and left ventricle and its accentuation in late diastole by atrial contraction in patients in sinus rhythm. Finally, the loud first heart sound is contributed by the fibrosis of the leaflets and is lost with leaflet calcification. Many patients with mitral stenosis have some degree of mitral regurgitation which is not significant in the presence of severe stenosis. In the presence of pulmonary hypertension, the second heart sound is usually loud and the jugular venous pressure is raised. In patients with significant tricuspid regurgitation, whether secondary to pulmonary hypertension or due to rheumatic tricuspid valve, there is clear V-wave in the jugular venous pulse followed by a deep Y descent and expansile pulsation of the liver. The murmur of tricuspid regurgitation is not usually prominent, particularly when it is severe.

Investigations

Chest X-ray and electrocardiogram: Early in the disease process, a chest X-ray may show completely normal cardiac silhouette. Later, as the disease progresses, left atrial enlargement appears and a prominent left atrial appendage contour may become very evident. Left atrial double-density and elevation of left main bronchus may also be evident. In patients with raised left atrial pressure, pulmonary vascular redistribution 'dilated upper lobe veins' and interstitial pulmonary edema 'Kerley B lines' may be seen. The central pulmonary arteries become prominent as pulmonary hypertension develops, and upper lobe deviation is also seen. Finally, the right-sided dilatation may be seen as tricuspid regurgitation develops. The electrocardiogram shows a broad and notched P-wave, due to left atrial hypertrophy, as a classical finding in mitral stenosis 'P mitrale'. Patients with atrial fibrillation show clear electrocardiographic signs of irregular narrow QRS.

Echocardiography: Echocardiography is the investigation of choice in mitral valve disease. A typical picture of rheumatic valve disease is a short fibrosed and stiff posterior leaflet, fibrosed anterior leaflet that bows down towards the ventricle in diastole and narrow valve area. Short axis images clearly demonstrate the fused commissures. Also, 2D images show the extent of chordal fibrosis, shortage and the inflow tract. Other associated abnormalities are clearly seen and quantitatively assessed by echocardiography. Left atrial diameter, area and volume are measured from frozen images and used as a criterion for anti-coagulation therapy. Tricuspid valve anatomy and function should always be assessed in patients with rheumatic mitral valve disease. Two-dimensional images and Doppler velocities also assist in confirming the diagnosis of organic tricuspid valve disease. The same principle applies to organic rheumatic aortic valve leaflets, which are not infrequently seen in this setting. Color flow Doppler demonstrates the presence and severity of valve regurgitation. Finally, right heart size and function should be studied as an integral part of the echocardiographic examination of such patients. The severity of pulmonary hypertension is quantified from the continuous wave Doppler recording of the tricuspid regurgitation using the modified Bernoulli equation P(pressure)$=4V$ (velocity)^2. Patients with unexplained fluid retention should have right-sided heart physiology assessed in great detail which should guide towards optimum patient management. Severe tricuspid regurgitation on color and continuous wave Doppler should be differentiated from restrictive right ventricular physiology as a cause for fluid retention. While severe tricuspid regurgitation presents with V-wave on JVP and systolic flow reversal in SVC and IVC, restrictive RV disease is associated with deep Y descent on JVP and early diastolic flow in the venae cava.

Assessment of Mitral Stenosis Severity

Mitral Valve Area

In order to gain a flow-independent measure of the degree of narrowing, mitral valve area is frequently calculated. A number of methods have been proposed for this but none is entirely satisfactory. There is no agreed gold standard against which non-invasive measures can be calibrated, and when compared with one another, correlation coefficients are usually too low to be applicable in individual patients. Furthermore, it is questionable whether the complex hemodynamic disturbance to atrioventricular flow can be summed up in a simple statement of area.

a) *Planimetry*: It involves tracing the inner border of the mitral valve opening in diastole obtained from the short axis view. This has been shown to correlate with valve area measured by catheterization [11]. It has its limitations, particularly in the presence of significant leaflet tip calcification, poor border detection and varying degrees of opening time due to atrial fibrillation Figure 1.5.

b) *Vena contracta*: The width of color flow jet (vena contracta) in two orthogonal planes correlates with planimetry-estimated values of mitral valve area [12] Figure 1.6.

c) *Flow convergence (proximal isovelocity area—PISA)*: Blood flow through a narrowed orifice converges in a series of proximal isovelocity hemispheres (isovelocity surface area). In mitral stenosis, it can be demonstrated by mosaic color Doppler on the atrial side in diastole. The flow rate is calculated by $2\pi r^2 v$, where r is the distance to a contour of velocity v, defined by the change in color at the aliasing boundary Figure 1.6. The narrowed orifice area can be calculated by dividing peak flow rate by maximal velocity through the orifice (obtained from the continuous wave Doppler). Mitral valve area calculated by this method has been shown to correlate with that obtained by

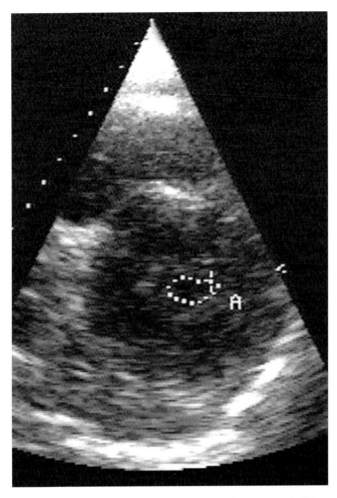

FIGURE 1.5. Parasternal short axis view of a rheumatic mitral valve showing a traced valve area of 1.0 cm^2.

conventional catheterization. However, flow convergence method is subject to geometric complexities of the mitral valve orifice [13].

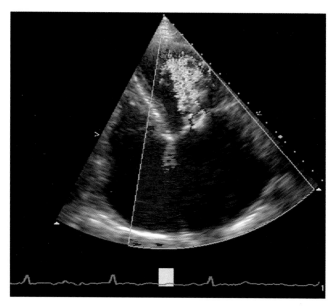

FIGURE 1.6. Transmitral flow convergence velocities from a patient with mitral stenosis. Note the change in velocity before the stenotic orifice.

d) *Transmitral pressure drop*: Using modified Bernoulli equation ($4V^2$) peak and minimum mitral pressure drop can be measured and mean value calculated [14] **Figure 1.7**.

e) *Pressure ½ time*: This is the time taken by the early diastolic transmitral pressure to drop to ½ its peak value (or the time taken for initial velocity divided by square root of 2 which is 1.4). Mitral area is then calculated as a constant (220) divided by pressure ½ time. **Figure 1.8** although mitral pressure ½ time has been found to correlate with invasively measured mitral valve area, it too has major limitations, particularly in patients with atrial fibrillation and fast heart rate. Also pressure ½ time depends on the left ventricular inflow resistance due to the funnel shape of the mitral apparatus including both orifice and subvalvar component. More resistance at the subval-

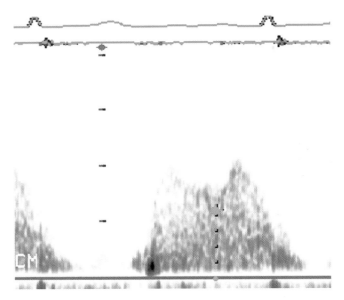

FIGURE 1.7. Transmitral forward flow velocities by CW Doppler, showing raised early diastolic pressure drop component giving a mean of 8 mmHg.

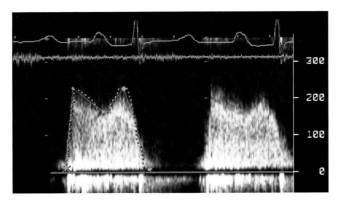

FIGURE 1.8. Transmitral Doppler flow velocities from a patient with mitral stenosis showing pressure $\frac{1}{2}$ time measurement.

var apparatus may slow the pressure decline across the inflow tract, so that pressure $\frac{1}{2}$ time is usually smaller than that obtained from 2D planimetry. The opposite is seen in patients with concomitant aortic regurgitation or left ventricular hypertrophy, when pressure $\frac{1}{2}$ time overestimates the degree of mitral stenosis. It may, therefore, provide unreliable values after mitral valvuloplasty. The main reason for underestimating the accuracy of this method is the fact that it relies on the pressure fall which is frequently not exponential [15, 16].

f) *Continuity equation*: It is based on the principle of mass and energy conservation. The flow at all points along a tube is constant and equals the product of mean velocity and cross-sectional area. Mitral valve area is calculated as the product of aortic or pulmonary annular cross-sectional area and the ratio of the respective valve velocity time integral to that of the mitral stenotic continuous wave velocity. Although a more complex approach, this method is preferable in patients with additional significant aortic regurgitation in whom pressure $\frac{1}{2}$ time overestimates mitral valve area [17].

Mitral valve area >1.5 cm^2 is usually considered as mild stenosis, between 1.0 and 1.5 cm^2 as moderate and <1 cm^2 as severe stenosis.

The common practice now is to study most patients with significant mitral valve disease by transesophageal echocardiography since it provides more detailed assessment of the mitral valve, subvalvar apparatus and the presence of left atrial spontaneous contrast and appendage clots. Mitral valve area measurements can also be obtained from transesophageal images as described above Figure 1.9.

Cardiac catheterization: Echocardiography has replaced cardiac catheterization in making the diagnosis of mitral stenosis. Cardiac catheterization may only provide additional information on pulmonary vascular resistance and coronary artery disease before surgery.

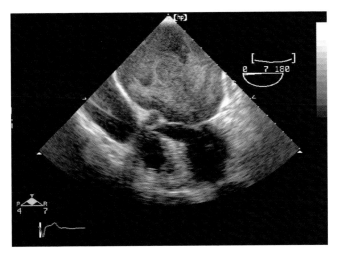

FIGURE 1.9. Transesophageal echocardiogram from a patient with severe rheumatic mitral stenosis, dilated left atrium and spontaneous echo-contrast.

Disease Progress

There is a significant time lag between the acute event of rheumatic fever and the presentation of mitral stenosis with mild symptoms, which could be up to 15 years. Patients may need another 10 years to develop signs and symptoms of severe stenosis. The likely reason behind this delay is the time needed for rheumatic leaflet fibrosis and calcification to develop and cause raised left atrial pressure. This time lag between acute rheumatic fever and clinical presentation varies significantly between the West and developing countries. While in Europe and North America patients need valve surgery for mitral stenosis in their fifties, those in developing countries need it in their thirties [18]. Also the clinical outcome of patients with unoperated rheumatic mitral stenosis has changed significantly over time, with 20-year follow-up mortality dropping from historically 85% to recently 44%, in those who refuse surgery [19].

Treatment

Medical therapy: The only medical treatment in mitral stenosis is the prophylactic measures against rheumatic fever, endocarditis and diuretics for raised left atrial pressure. There is no medication that has a direct effect on slowing disease progress.

Follow-up: Patients with mitral stenosis are followed up clinically using non-invasive investigations, particularly Doppler echocardiography. The frequency of follow-up is tailored according to individual patient's clinical condition and the severity of mitral valve disease. While it could be every 2 years in a patient with mild stenosis and regurgitation it needs a shorter period of follow-up in another with severe stenosis and evidence of pulmonary hypertension. A closer follow-up should be devised for pregnant women who have mitral stenosis.

Interventional Treatment

Early intervention in the disease process before the development of atrial fibrillation and enlarged left atrium is highly recommended, provided a conservative procedure is possible. In patients who develop atrial fibrillation attempts to restore sinus rhythm are usually unsuccessful unless associated with surgery. To maintain sinus rhythm, the organic mitral lesion should be dealt with either interventionally or surgically. In addition to heart rate control, digoxin may keep patients with modestly dilated left atrium in sinus rhythm. Once atrial fibrillation is organized attention should be diverted to rate control with digoxin, β-blockers or calcium channel blockers. With persistent atrial fibrillation anti-coagulants are essential and INR level should be monitored and maintained at 2.5–3.5. Patients recommended for percutaneous mitral valvoplasty should receive stable anti-coagulation therapy for at least 3 months before procedure and transesophageal echo should exclude left atrial clot. Those who need surgical intervention may receive a Maze procedure as a means for restoring sinus rhythm. This involves surgically creating a single electrical pathway from the sinus node to the AV node while isolating the abnormal electrical activity of the left and right atrial tissues. Recently, electrophysiological mapping with isolation of pulmonary veins has offered an alternative procedure [20]. The success of Maze procedure varies significantly, ranging between 25 and 80% [21] even after an initially successful procedure.

I. valvuloplasty

This technique uses a percutaneous catheter double balloon or Inoue balloon valvuloplasty. It is only recommended when mitral valve leaflets are pliable and there is no valve calcification including the subvalvar apparatus. Left atrial clot should be excluded by transesophageal echo. The increase in mitral valve area occurs along the plan of commissures and results in increased opening angle provided there is no calcification. An echocardiographic (Abascal) score is used to morphologically assess mitral valve structure and function [22–24]. Assigning a score ranging from 0 to 4 to each of mitral leaflet mobility, thickening, calcification and subvalvular thickening provides a numerical assessment of overall valve function. The higher the score, the more anatomically deformed and functionally abnormal the valve, hence the likelihood of poor outcome after balloon valvuloplasty. Mid- and long-term results of the procedure in well-selected cases are promising. A successful procedure is judged by >50% increase in mitral valve area. This can be underestimated early after procedure because of the iatrogenically created left to right shunt across the atrial septum. The latter results from the guide wire insertion through the atrial septum. This shunt has been reported to disappear within 6 months after the procedure. Significant mitral regurgitation may occur in >30% of patients after balloon valvuloplasty. It is usually more severe when

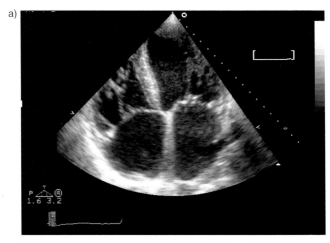

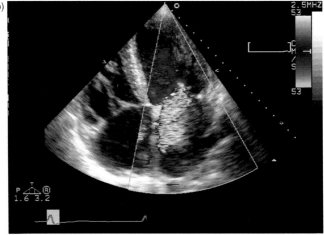

FIGURE 1.10. Apical views from a patient with rheumatic mitral valve leaflets after balloon valvuloplasty demonstrating significant regurgitation and atrial shunt across the mid-septum.

the procedure is complicated by a tear in one of the two leaflets. Figure 1.10 Transesophageal echocardiography is of particular importance before and during this procedure in order to

   i. assess valve structure and calcification before procedure,

  ii. exclude left atrial appendage or free wall thrombus,

 iii. guide the way during septal puncture,

 iv. ascertain balloon position across the valve orifice,

  v. assess pressure drop and mitral valve area after each inflation,

 vi. detect early complication, i.e. leaflet tear, ruptured chordae or mitral regurgitation that needs urgent intervention,

vii. confirm any perforation of left atrial free wall,

viii. assess left to right shunt.

II. Surgery

For symptomatic cases not suitable for valvuloplasty, surgery is the only alternative.

a) *Closed mitral valvotomy*: This is appropriate for young patients who are in sinus rhythm, with no other valve disease, in whom mitral valve leaflets are mobile and not calcified. This is an underrated operation, and up to 40-year follow-up results are exceptionally good. This historical procedure aims at opening the mitral valve by applying a dilator through the ventricular apex and feeling the valve leaflets and orifice by the surgeon's finger until the desired valve area is achieved. The first successful operations were carried out in 1948. This operation has been intensively used in the UK and other countries with an average mortality of 3–4% [25].

b) *Open valvotomy*: This operation requires the use of an extracorporeal circulation and aims at direct visualization of the mitral valve through a medial sternotomy or smaller incisions such as a right anterior thoracotomy and involves careful dissection of the fused commissures under direct vision. In contrast to the closed operation, the surgeon is able to deal with the subvalvar apparatus, the fused chordae and correction of chordal shortening, if required. The left atrial appendage can also be visualized and if there is thrombus present it can be removed. With appropriate patient selection and pre-operative evaluation, open commissurotomy is feasible in most patients, with an operative mortality of approximately 1% [26]. Correction of associated rheumatic mitral regurgitation in some cases has been recently undertaken. Open mitral valvotomy can also be performed with computerized robotic technology via 3–4 ports in the chest wall.

c) *Mitral valve replacement*: This procedure is required in pure mitral stenosis when the valve is heavily calcified. It involves either a mechanical (St Jude Medical) or a tissue valve (bioprosthesis) substitute with very good long-term follow-up. Despite that, surgical mortality for mitral valve replacement varies according to other co-morbidities. While it is in the order of 3% in patients with isolated mitral valve stenosis it could be as high as 12% in patients with additional pulmonary hypertension. Cryopreserved mitral homografts have been proposed recently [27] as a better option. Although this operation has significant theoretical advantages including better longevity, lack of need for anti-coagulants in patients with sinus rhythm and achieving a low forward gradient, this remains an innovative procedure with a mortality of 25–50% of failing valves within 3 years of implantation [28]. Finally, The use of a pulmonary autograft in a Dacron tube for mitral valve replacement has been proposed but the general experience is limited [29]. This technique (top-hat) could be ideal for patients who have limited access to anti-coagulation clinics, particularly in the developing countries. Traditional procedure of mitral valve replacement involves cutting the heads of the papillary muscles. This resulted in significant asynchrony of the left ventricle, particularly the long axis when its main shortening phase occurs in diastole rather than in systole Figure 1.11. The loss of longitudinal function renders the ventricle more spherical in diastole and hence has adverse implications on filling pattern and symptoms. The current surgical approach is to preserve the papillary muscles as much as possible. This change in procedural plan has resulted in maintained long axis function and improvement of ventricular hemodynamics and symptoms after surgery.

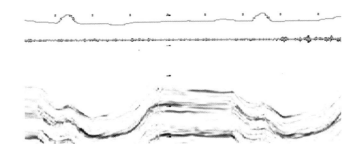

FIGURE 1.11. Long axis recording from left ventricular free wall of a patient after mitral valve replacement and cutting of papillary muscles. Note the marked incoordinate behavior and the extent of shortening that takes place in diastole rather than systole.

The Role of Echocardiography in Patient Selection for Surgery

1) *Assessing ventricular function*: In addition to valve assessment, transthoracic echo provides an exceptional means for quantifying ventricular function in these patients. Symptoms may result from poor ventricular function, whether caused by the rheumatic disease itself or an additional etiology, i.e., coronary artery disease. Raised end-diastolic pressure results in accentuated left ventricular filling pressures which is complicated by pulmonary venous congestion and hence development of dyspnea. Additional atrial fibrillation usually worsens the situation by losing the atrial filling component and compromises the stroke volume, particularly when fast. Such severely disturbed physiology should be excluded before qualifying mitral valve stenosis as the main cause of symptoms. Furthermore, ignoring such abnormalities before surgery may result in peri- or early post-operative complications with increased mortality.

2) *Degree of valve calcification*: Transesophageal echo provides additional details on the mitral valve and subvalvar

apparatus that may influence decision making. Pliable leaflets with mild calcification suggest valvotomy whereas extensive calcification requires valve replacement. Sub-valvar stenosis by fibrosed chordae and papillary muscles also favors valve replacement. Any evidence for additional endocarditis or possible complications such as 'shunt formation' can be dealt with at the time of surgery.

3) *Atrial fibrillation*: Patients with atrial fibrillation and a modestly dilated left atrium may be recommended for elective ablation of the pulmonary venous orifice at the time of mitral valve surgery. When such procedure is performed under transesophageal echo guidance, it may add to its rate of success. Left atrial clot, whether mural or in the atrial appendage, can also be decorticated during the procedure.

4) *Other valve disease*: Transthoracic echo provides quantitative assessment of aortic and tricuspid valve involvement, when combined with pulsed and continuous wave Doppler. If found, a balanced physiology should be considered when assessing more than one diseased valve, i.e., tricuspid stenosis tends to underestimate mitral stenosis, and mitral stenosis underestimates aortic stenosis. Transesophageal echo may add more clarity in assessing tricuspid valve anatomy in this condition.

Mitral Annular Calcification

Mitral annular calcification is usually a disease of the elderly, predominantly females. It is also present in other conditions such as hypertension and/or aortic stenosis. Calcification affects the heart either in a patchy manner or uniformly. It usually involves the mitral annulus but can extend into the basal septum, the aortic root and cusps or rarely the whole of the ventricular basal region. However, if the calcification encroaches on the basal part of the mitral leaflets it may result in increased filling velocities. It can be associated with mild mitral regurgitation but more commonly conduction disturbances occur in approximately 50% of patients. When affecting the mitral annulus, the leaflets themselves are usually spared, and the valve does not become stenotic Figure 1.12.

Management: In the absence of significant mitral stenosis, valve replacement is not indicated. When involving the aortic root and cusps leading to stenosis, aortic valve and root replacement is usually successful. Calcification of the mitral annulus is not superficial but it invades deeply into the myocardium. During surgery, decalcifying the mitral ring for valve replacement may result in myocardial perforation. Mitral valve replacement therefore should never be performed for pure mitral ring calcification.

Mitral Regurgitation

Mitral regurgitation results from abnormalities affecting components of the mitral valve: leaflets, annulus, chordae or papillary muscles. The causes are multiple in comparison to mitral stenosis. Myocardial disease when affecting particularly the basal part of the ventricle may result in various degrees of mitral regurgitation with the commonest cause—ischemic myocardial dysfunction. Less common causes of mitral regurgitation are mitral valve prolapse, myxomatous degeneration, endocarditis, non-ischemic dilated cardiomyopathy and other infiltrative disease and fibrosis.

Etiology of Mitral Regurgitation

A. Ischemic Mitral Regurgitation

The most common component of the mitral valve apparatus that is subject to ischemic dysfunction is the postero-medial papillary muscle which is also predisposed to infarction. This is because it is supplied by a single branch of the posterior descending artery and tends to have only a few

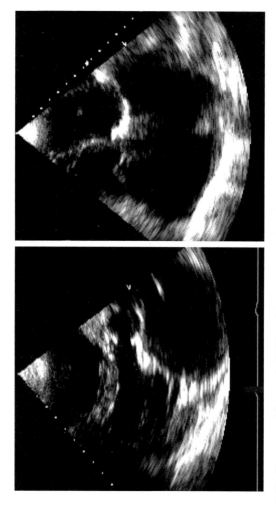

FIGURE 1.12. Parasternal long axis (left) and four chamber (right) views of the left heart showing a heavily calcified mitral annulus and normal leaflets.

collaterals. The antero-lateral papillary muscle receives blood from branches of both the left anterior descending artery and the circumflex artery so it is less susceptible to ischaemia. Ischaemic disturbances of left ventricular function contribute to the development of mitral regurgitation through a number of mechanisms: (a) regional wall motion abnormalities with adverse ventricular remodeling and systolic tenting of the valve leaflets, (b) left ventricular dilatation and shape change that alters normal alignment of the papillary muscles and results in leaflet tethering and inadequate closure and (c) annular dilatation that leads to inadequate annular contraction and leaflet coaption. These mechanisms may contribute to further enlargement of the left ventricle and deterioration of its function which itself would add to the severity of mitral regurgitation. Four clinical presentations are seen in ischaemic mitral regurgitation: (i) acute myocardial infarction, (ii) papillary muscle rupture, (iii) reversible ischaemic myocardial dysfunction in the presence of preserved left ventricular systolic function and (iv) end-stage ischaemic cardiomyopathy with reduced function.

Acute myocardial infarction: Mitral regurgitation is common in acute myocardial infarction and significant regurgitation complicates up to 15% of cases. Although most such cases present within the context of acute myocardial infarction, some may present with acute development of mitral regurgitation [30]. Most patients presenting with myocardial infarction complicated by mitral regurgitation have right and circumflex coronary artery disease that causes inferior wall dysfunction. Mitral regurgitation therefore does not seem to be related to the infarct size but the extent of ischaemic dysfunction and involvement of postero-medial papillary muscle. The resulting poor support to the posterior leaflet, referred to as tethering, causes lack of leaflet coaption and valve incompetence. When severe mitral regurgitation develops it carries poor prognosis with mortality rising up to 25% at 30 days and over 50% at 1 year [31]. The effect of myocardial reperfusion on mitral regurgitation remains controversial.

Papillary muscle rupture: Although a rare complication to myocardial infarction, complete papillary muscle rupture causes severe mitral regurgitation and cardiogenic shock which is usually fatal, 70% within 24 hours without emergency surgery. Surgical repair of the papillary muscle is not feasible in most cases because of the extent of the necrotic tissue [32] so valve replacement is necessary and its risk is influenced by other factors including severe left ventricular dysfunction which usually exists. Papillary muscle rupture occurs 2–5 days after the onset of the infarct. Incomplete rupture, usually of only one head of the papillary muscle, occurs 4–5 days after the infarct with gradual deterioration of mitral regurgitation. This increases pre-existing left ventricular dysfunction Figure 1.13.

Ischaemic mitral regurgitation in a normal left ventricle: Patients with long-standing ischaemic myocardial dysfunction may have exertional reversible ischaemia. If this affects the posterior wall of the left ventricle it leads to further deterioration of posterior wall function and consequently the posterior leaflet function and the development of mitral regurgitation. Exertional breathlessness in these patients does not always have to be due to raised end-diastolic pressure but a sudden increase in left atrial pressure by the development of mitral regurgitation with exercise, particularly in those with dilated left atrium and those with poor atrial compliance. Stress echocardiography is ideal for demonstrating the ischaemic ventricular dysfunction and the development of mitral regurgitation and raised left atrial pressure, hence the beneficial role of anti-anginal therapy and afterload reduction. Patients who develop significant mitral regurgitation with stress who are accepted for coronary artery bypass graft surgery should receive mitral valve repair, a ring insertion, at the same time of surgical revascularization [33] to avoid potential persistent symptoms despite successful surgery.

Ischaemic mitral regurgitation in ventricular dysfunction: Mitral regurgitation is very common in patients with long-standing ischaemic left ventricular dysfunction and those in

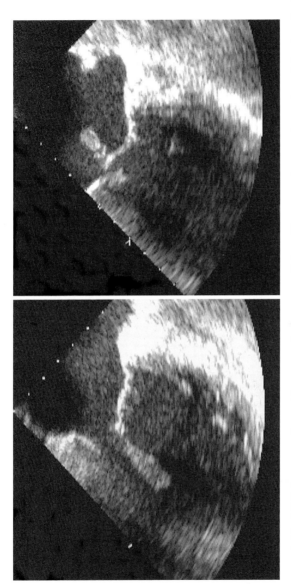

FIGURE 1.13. TOE from a patient with ruptured postero-medial papillary muscle. Note bouncing of the detached segment into the left atrium in systole.

end stage ventricular disease. Since, in these patients, valve leaflets appear morphologically normal, the mitral regurgitation is described as 'functional'. Three-dimensional echocardiographic assessment of the mitral valve proves that the valve itself is not entirely normal, with long-standing progressive changes in the interleaflet relations and subvalvar apparatus. Reducing ventricular pressures may improve left ventricular geometry and lowering blood pressure may reduce mitral regurgitation severity.

Pathophysiology of Mitral Regurgitation

Regurgitant orifice and jet: The regurgitant volume of mitral regurgitation is calculated as the regurgitant flow over the regurgitant area. The flow velocity through the orifice is related to the ventricular–atrial systolic pressure difference. High left ventricular systolic pressures, e.g., systemic hypertension, increase mitral regurgitation volume and low left ventricular pressure reduces it. Left atrial pressure in acute mitral regurgitation is raised with a V-wave in late systole due to the increased volume and the velocity of blood entering the left atrium. The absence of a V-wave on the left atrial pressure recording or pulmonary wedge pressure, however, does not exclude the diagnosis of severe mitral regurgitation. With severe mitral regurgitation, the raised retrograde stroke volume into the left atrium causes increased forward flow across the mitral valve into the left ventricle which increases ventricular activity and the rate of increase of cavity size. Mitral regurgitation is often a dynamic lesion and the size of the regurgitant orifice and regurgitant volume may vary with the pressure gradient across the valve and with changes in left ventricular volume and geometry. The effective regurgitant orifice area itself may increase with significantly abnormal ventricular geometry. Thus, successful reduction of left ventricular volume by optimum medical therapy or pacing and improvement of its systolic function may assist in reducing severity of mitral regurgitation and opening the vicious circle.

Afterload: Mitral regurgitation is an isolated volume overload on the left ventricle. It provides the physiological equivalent of afterload reduction so that a normal forward cardiac output is maintained by the combination of increased ejection fraction and higher pre-load. Therefore, unlike the pressure overload in mitral regurgitation the coronary blood flow is normal and the increase in myocardial oxygen consumption is only minimum.

The left atrium: Left atrial volume increases in patients with mitral regurgitation in response to the increase in its pressure [34]. The other mechanism behind the increase in left atrial volume is the transmission of the mitral regurgitation kinetic energy to the left atrial wall as well as the development of atrial fibrillation. These effects balance those of mitral regurgitation jet on the left atrial pressure which is normal in compensated patients. Although the atrial size is increased in mitral regurgitation, the risk of thrombus formation is much less than that seen in mitral stenosis because of the fast regurgitant jet that speeds the atrial blood circulation[35].

The right heart: The risk of right heart disease and dysfunction in mitral regurgitation is very similar to that in mitral stenosis. The raised left atrial pressure and pulmonary venous pressure are directly reflected on right ventricular systolic pressure and hence eventual right ventricular hypertrophy and dilatation. Patients with coronary artery disease and right ventricular involvement may present with enlarged and impaired right ventricular cavity, irrespective of the severity of mitral regurgitation.

B. Mitral Valve Prolapse

Mitral valve prolapse is a genetic connective tissue disorder that affects the mitral leaflets, chordae and annulus with an autosomal dominant pattern of inheritance and variable penetrance [36]. The specific gene defect for mitral prolapse has not yet been identified. The suspicion of mitral prolapse is raised by identification of mid to late systolic click and late systolic murmur. The mid systolic click corresponds to the sudden posterior movement of one or both leaflets towards the left atrium. Mitral prolapse can be classified into two types: benign one, seen in the young, commonly women which does not always progress, and the myxomatous leaflet disease, seen in the elderly—'myxomatous mitral valve disease'. In general, significant mitral regurgitation is very common in myxomatous leaflet disease and needs surgical repair. The exact genetic and natural history difference between the two conditions is not yet clear but almost 2–6% of adults have some degree of mitral leaflet prolapse [37]. Although the morphology of the mitral valve leaflets varies between patients, in general severe mitral regurgitation is associated with redundant leaflets, longer posterior leaflet and a larger annulus. Chordal distribution may also be abnormal in mitral prolapse which may be a relative scarcity of chordae attached to the central scallop of the posterior leaflet, increased chordal division [38] or a higher incidence of chordal rupture. The commonest site for posterior mitral prolapse is the middle scallop (P2). Histologically, the leaflets show thickening of the spongiosa and disruption of the fibrosa with fragmentation [39]. Leaflet collagen is also abnormal with high rate of synthesis, deficiency in collagen 3 and splitting of collagen with fiber disarray [40]. Finally, a defect in a gene encoding a component of microfibrils similar to Marfan syndrome might be another etiology for mitral prolapse.

Clinical Presentation

Symptoms: Patients with mitral prolapse may live for years unidentified until incidentally examined and the click and the mitral regurgitation murmur are heard, indicating mild mitral regurgitation. Those with severe regurgitation may present with dyspnea or arrhythmia. The most common symptoms are atypical chest pain, palpitations, dyspnea, fatigue and dizziness which are not specific and do not always guide towards the differential diagnosis of mitral prolapse. Echocardiography is the mainstay in making an accurate quantitative diagnosis of mitral regurgitation and in identifying the exact cause for it.

Physical examination: The cardinal signs of mild mitral prolapse are the mid systolic click due to the backward movement of the mitral leaflet into the left atrium and the late systolic mitral regurgitation which occurs after the click. As mitral regurgitation becomes severe, the characteristics of the murmur change and it becomes early systolic and short in duration. The loudness of the murmur correlates with the regurgitant severity and a systolic thrill is usually associated with severe regurgitation. Murmurs less than grade 2/6 indicate mild regurgitation. With acute mitral regurgitation no murmur may be audible. The radiation of the murmur depends on the direction of the regurgitant jet. A posterolateral jet seen in ischaemic mitral regurgitation, anterior leaflet disease and dilated cardiomyopathy radiates from the apex to the axilla and even to the back. An antero-superior jet due to posterior leaflet prolapse is heard better at the lower left sternal edge or cardiac base and even on the carotids. Other physical signs depend on the severity of mitral regurgitation and possible complications, e.g., pulmonary hypertension. With severe mitral regurgitation patients may present with atrial fibrillation. Compared with normal individuals, patients with mitral prolapse have a higher prevalence of endocarditis, 43% compared to 13%.

Investigations

Echocardiography: Two-dimensional echocardiography provides a thorough assessment of the anatomy and function of mitral valve leaflets. A clear understanding of the three dimensionality of the mitral valve assists in obtaining detailed information on the behavior of each of the two leaflets in various views from transthoracic and transesophageal examinations. The echocardiographic criterion for mitral prolapse is the presence of at least 2 mm systolic displacement of the leaflets beyond the mitral annular plan. Severe myxomatous degeneration is associated with thickening of the leaflets and the appearance of extensive folding or redundancy of the leaflets in diastole, chordal elongation and systolic anterior motion of the leaflets. Secondary mitral prolapse can easily be distinguished from primary prolapse, e.g., in cases like Marfan syndrome where the leaflets are thin and long and tend to prolapse, particularly the anterior one. Similar pathology may be seen in hypertrophic cardiomyopathy with long leaflets and systolic anterior motion of the mitral valve. In addition to leaflet examination echocardiography provides clear information on the mitral valve apparatus, annular diameter, left ventricular size and function as well as left atrial size and pulmonary artery pressure. Due to its non-invasive nature, it is ideal in the follow-up of such patients in order to identify early deterioration of regurgitation severity or ventricular dysfunction as an indication for a need for surgical repair. Patients recommended for surgical repair need detailed transthoracic and transesophageal echocardiographic assessment of the anatomy of the valve and subvalvular apparatus which should assist surgeons to plan their procedure ahead.

Natural History and Complications

Overall survival in patients with mitral prolapse accounts for 97% at 6 years and 88% at 8 years [41]. Patients with myxomatous mitral valve disease and a flail leaflet have a 10-year survival of only 10% [42]. With posterior leaflet myxomatous prolapse, progressive chronic mitral regurgitation is associated with progressive radial dilatation of the left atrium and left ventricle [43]. Leaflet prolapse caused by ruptured chordae may cause only mild mitral regurgitation with a stable clinical course for years with no further deterioration. Significant mitral regurgitation occurs in less than 10% of patients with posterior prolapse compared to 25% of those with anterior leaflet prolapse. In contrast, the incidence of atrial fibrillation and heart failure is significantly higher in posterior leaflet prolapse compared to anterior leaflet prolapse. Overall, irrespective of the etiology of leaflet disease left ventricular dysfunction, presented by increased end-systolic diameter, as well as right ventricular dysfunction, as a complication of pulmonary hypertension, are the two most important determinants of outcome.

There is a clear relationship between mitral valve prolapse, arrhythmia and sudden death [44]. The annual rate of sudden death in mitral prolapse is approximately 2%, which significantly falls after surgical repair. Controversy exists with regard to the relationship between mitral prolapse and embolic events. However, it is generally accepted that patients with severe mitral regurgitation carry much less risk from thromboembolism compared to those with mild regurgitation and dilated atria, irrespective of the presence of atrial fibrillation. The risk of endocarditis in mitral prolapse is estimated at 3–8 times that of the general population. The underlying mechanism is the leaflet prolapse that causes significant turbulence of the blood flow across the valve orifice which disrupts the platelets and fibrin deposition on the valve surface and creates a good substrate for potential superimposed secondary infection.

Management of Mitral Valve Prolapse

Strict echocardiographic criteria are crucial for making accurate diagnosis which includes the leaflet thickness, redundancy and the presence of systolic displacement of the leaflets into the left atrium and resulting mitral regurgitation. Transthoracic echocardiography is perfectly adequate for this purpose but transesophageal echo provides more details on the valve anatomy and other potential complications, e.g., left atrial thrombus. Screening of first degree family members demonstrates similar disease in approximately 30% of cases [45]. Even in the absence of significant mitral regurgitation, identifying such individuals is important for strict antibiotic prophylaxis.

Follow-up: Patients with chronic mitral regurgitation may survive for a long time with no limiting symptoms. Once symptoms develop they suggest a serious need for surgical correction of the valve regurgitation in order to avoid irreversible left ventricular dysfunction. Assessment of such patients during routine follow-up identifies those likely to need surgical intervention even in the absence of symptoms. While patients with acute regurgitation secondary to papillary muscle rupture need emergency surgery this does not necessarily apply to those with ruptured chordae or chronic ischaemic regurgitation. Patients need to be stabilized and other risk factors and co-morbidities identified and optimally managed before surgery. An increase in severity of mitral regurgitation with or without complications suggests a need for surgical intervention.

Medical therapy: There is no medical therapy that cures mitral valve prolapse. However, endocarditis prophylaxis is a very strong recommendation [46]. In the absence of mitral regurgitation, isolated mitral prolapse might not be counted as a serious indication. Symptomatic supra-ventricular arrhythmia needs optimum therapy by beta-blockers. Patients with ventricular tachycardia and syncope should be evaluated for implantable defibrillator, using acceptable criteria. Those in atrial fibrillation should be given anti-coagulants and INR adjusted at 2.5–3.5.

C. Dilated Cardiomyopathy

Mitral regurgitation is also common in dilated non-ischaemic cardiomyopathy. Dilatation of the left ventricle disturbs the normal closure of the mitral valve; the leaflets fail to coapt and hence mitral regurgitation. The benefit of surgical intervention and ring insertion in these patients remains controversial [47]. Appropriate pacing for dilated cardiomyopathy has been reported to reduce the severity of mitral regurgitation [48]. Medical treatment of patients with dilated cardiomyopathy should be carefully tailored. Vasodilators improve prognosis and also reduce pre-load and the venous return which improves leaflet coaption and reduces mitral regurgitation. Their effect on the afterload improves the forward flow and reduces the retrograde flow across the mitral valve. Carvedilol has been shown to improve left ventricular shape by reducing its long axis length over diameter ratio 'cardiac index' and hence reducing mitral regurgitation severity [49]. Similar findings have been documented in patients receiving ACE-inhibitors or angiotensin receptor antagonist [50].

Assessment of Mitral Regurgitation Severity

The major determinant of mitral regurgitation severity is the effective regurgitant area, which may be fixed in rheumatic mitral valve disease, bacterial endocarditis and mitral prolapse. A regurgitant volume of 40 ml signifies a regurgitant fraction (volume of blood regurgitated into the left atrium) of 40% and regurgitant area (mitral valve incompetent area in systole) of 40 mm^2 [51].

a) *Large LV stroke volume*: An increase in left ventricular end-diastolic dimension and fall of end-systolic dimension suggest an overloaded ventricle and significant mitral regurgitation [52]. In this condition, fractional shortening and calculated ejection fraction should not be taken as measures of ventricular function. Absolute end-systolic diameter or volume is considered more accurate markers of ventricular disease. An end-systolic diameter >40 mm suggests independent left ventricular disease, the reversibility of which cannot be confirmed [53] Figure 1.14.

b) *Color flow area*: This is the most widely used technique. Maximum jet areas traced in different views correlate with severity of mitral regurgitation assessed by left

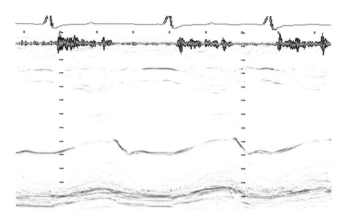

FIGURE 1.14.   M-mode of LV minor axis from a patient with severe mitral regurgitation. Note the relative difference between end-diastolic and end-systolic measurements and the rapid increase in early diastolic dimension due to severe mitral regurgitation.

ventriculography. A regurgitant area of $>8\,\mathrm{cm^2}$ or relative area $>40\%$ that of the left atrium suggests severe regurgitation, whereas a jet area of $<4\,\mathrm{cm^2}$ or relative area $<20\%$ identifies mild mitral regurgitation. This method relies on the clear display of a uniform regurgitant jet. If used alone, it may over or underestimate the regurgitation severity, particularly when the valve leaflets are flail and the jet uniformity is disrupted. Jet areas studied by transesophageal technique also tend to over estimate valve regurgitation [54–56] Figure 1.15.

c) *Proximal isovelocity surface area (PISA)*: As discussed in mitral stenosis, the regurgitant orifice area can be calculated by dividing peak flow rate by maximal velocity through the orifice (obtained from the continuous wave Doppler). A regurgitant orifice $>0.5\,\mathrm{cm^2}$ corresponds to a regurgitant fraction of $>50\%$ and thus signifies severe mitral regurgitation that needs surgery. Accurate measurements of flow convergence seem more reliable than color flow area mapping. However, flow convergence

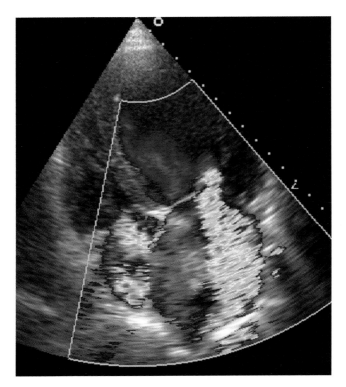

FIGURE 1.15. Apical four chamber view from a patient with severe mitral regurgitation on color Doppler. Note the absolute and relative differences in the regurgitant area with respect to that of the left atrium.

method is subject to geometric complexities of the regurgitant orifice that requires correction factors as in eccentric jets commonly seen in mitral valve prolapse Figure 1.16.

d) *Vena contracta*: Vena contracta is measured as the narrowest cross-sectional area of the mitral regurgitation jet at the level of the regurgitant orifice. The width of vena contracta has been found to correlate with the regurgitant volume; a width of 5 mm with a regurgitant volume of 60 ml suggests severe and a width <3 mm is consistent

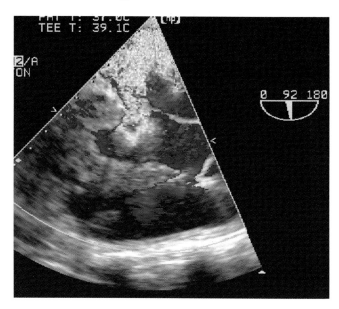

FIGURE 1.16. Color flow Doppler from a patient with severe mitral regurgitation. Note the aliasing velocities proximal to the valve orifice (on the ventricular side).

with mild mitral regurgitation. Vena contracta has been suggested to be independent of haemodynamic variables, orifice geometry and instrument setting and is associated with a low interobserver variability [57]. These advantages, however, do not apply to all patients, depending on the clarity of the jet (Figure 1.17).

e) *Systolic flow reversal in pulmonary veins*: This sign is helpful in determining regurgitant severity only when the jet is not eccentric. It is not of great use in patients with severe left ventricular disease in whom the systolic component of pulmonary venous flow is already poor and those with eccentric mitral regurgitation jet, e.g., posterior leaflet prolapse. Moreover, systolic flow in pulmonary veins is also affected by left atrial compliance, age and rhythm [58] Figure 1.18.

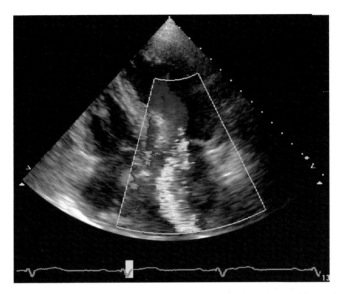

FIGURE 1.17. Apical four chamber view from a patient with moderate mitral regurgitation showing vena contracta of 4 mm.

f) *Continuous wave Doppler*: Mild mitral regurgitation usually stops well beyond (>80 ms) end-ejection corresponding to the left ventricular pressure decline during isovolumic relaxation period. A short deceleration limb of the retrograde transmitral signal (<40 ms beyond end-ejection) suggests significant regurgitation. Left ventricular–left atrial pressure equalization at end-ejection is consistent with severe mitral regurgitation. As left atrial pressure increases, the retrograde pressure drop across the mitral valve falls and no longer represents left ventricular systolic pressure. Left atrial pressure can be estimated as the transmitral retrograde pressure drop deducted from systolic blood pressure, particularly when it is low [59] Figure 1.19.

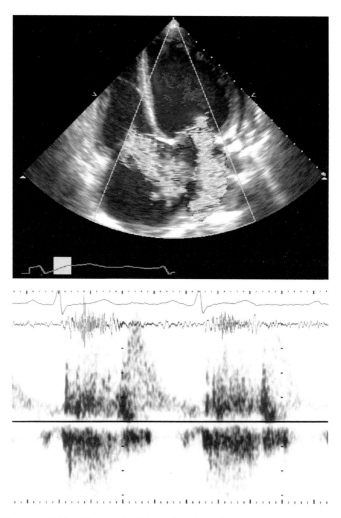

FIGURE 1.18. *Top*: Apical four chamber view from a patient with severe mitral regurgitation with the jet approaching the orifice of the pulmonary veins. *Bottom*: Pulsed wave velocity of the pulmonary venous flow from the same patient showing systolic flow reversal in the veins.

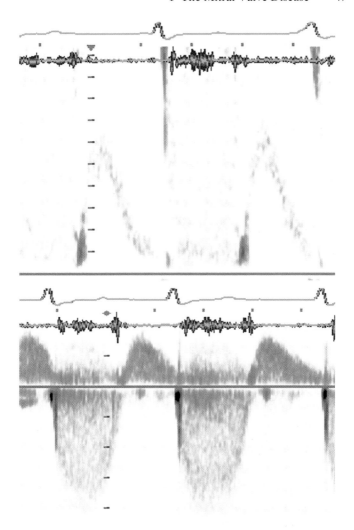

FIGURE 1.19. CW Doppler recording of severe mitral regurgitation and LV filling. Note the equalization of left atrial and left ventricular pressures in early diastole, ending retrograde flow at A2, short isovolumic relaxation time, and high LV filling velocities in early diastole.

g) *Left atrial emptying volume*: It is estimated as end-systolic volume–end-diastolic volume. A value of >40 ml identifies patients with severe mitral regurgitation [60].

h) *Continuity equation*: Relative aortic and mitral stroke volumes using the continuity equation, as previously discussed, determine regurgitation severity [61].

i) *Three-dimensional color Doppler*: It should always be considered that the mitral valve is a 3D structure and consequently its forward and retrograde flow jets. Despite the available techniques and their accuracy in determining mitral regurgitation severity each has its own limitations, because of the morphology of the regurgitant volume. Real time 3D echocardiography is now available and should provide more critical measures of jet severity. Published work so far has highlighted its potentials Figure 1.20.

Stress echocardiography: Symptomatic patients with no more than moderate mitral regurgitation, particularly caused by ischaemic etiology, should be studied by stress echocardiography. It assesses cardiac physiology and the stress-related change in mitral regurgitation severity at the time of symptom development. A drop in systolic blood pressure at fast heart rate is also taken as a marker of worsening regurgitation and compromised forward stroke volume. Patients with primarily left ventricular disease and incompliant cavity may develop raised left atrial pressure as a cause of their breathlessness, in the absence of significant mitral regurgitation. Thus, in such patients stress echocardiography may determine optimum management Figure 1.21.

Cardiac catheterization: In the presence of numerous means for non-invasive quantification of mitral regurgitation severity, invasive qualitative assessment is not now needed. Cardiac catheterization is only required to assess the coronary arteries in patients with unexplained left ventricular dysfunction and as a pre-operative procedure.

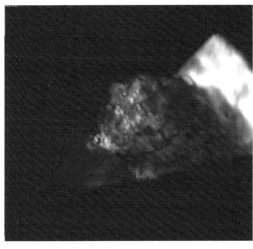

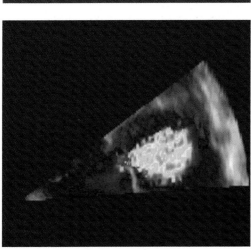

FIGURE 1.20. Three-dimension reconstruction of color Doppler mitral regurgitation (*right*) compared with its 2D images (*left*).

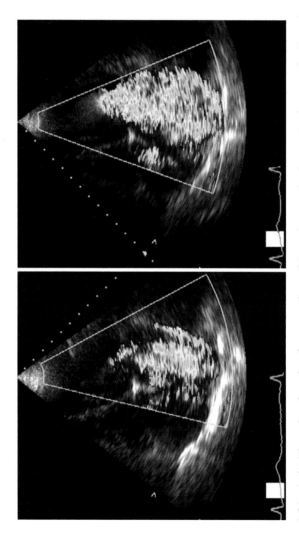

FIGURE 1.21. Apical four chamber view from a patient with moderate mitral regurgitation on color Doppler at rest (*left*) who developed severe valve incompetence at fast heart rate (*right*). Note the significant change in regurgitant area with stress.

Other Uncommon Causes of Mitral Regurgitation

a) Ruptured Chordae Tendineae

This is often a consequence of the myxomatous degeneration process that occurs with age. The development of significant mitral regurgitation is usually gradual. In some cases it takes an acute onset, particularly when it is not a complication of myxomatous degeneration, simply due to chordal rupture. The ventricle does not acutely dilate. The main symptoms are palpitations and dyspnea. Symptoms tend to improve over the course of the following weeks by which time the ventricle adapts itself to the volume load. Patients may present in intractable pulmonary edema in severe cases. This can be explained on the basis of long standing mitral regurgitation leading to a dilated and diseased ventricle. The combination of raised ventricular diastolic pressures and filling pressures worsens the condition and reduces the probabilities of having a possible successful repair [62, 63] Figure 1.22.

b) Endomyocardial Fibrosis

Endomyocardial fibrosis is an active process that involves the subendocardium and underlying myocardial layer. When affecting the right ventricle, it involves predominantly the apex, then progresses towards the tricuspid valve but spares the outflow tract. In the left ventricle, the inflow tract, apex and outflow tract are all involved. As the fibrosis affects the papillary muscle, it results in mitral and tricuspid valve regurgitation which can be severe enough to warrant valve replacement. This disease is common in the eastern part of Africa, South India and Brazil, and rarely affects Europeans. It is usually linked to hypereosinophilia due to helminthic infection Figure 1.23, 1.24.

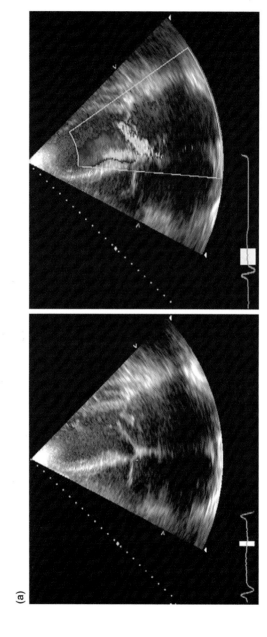

FIGURE 1.22. (**a**) Apical four chamber view from a patient with ruptured chordae resulting in posterior MV leaflet prolapse and MR.

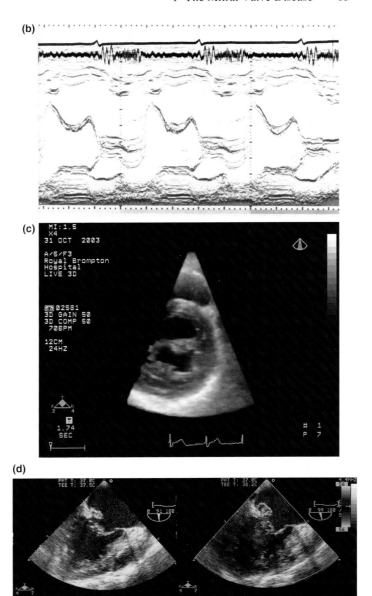

FIGURE 1.22. Continued.

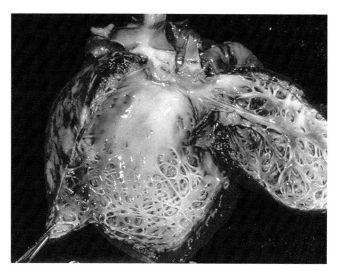

FIGURE 1.23. Pathology: dense pale fibrous tissue lining the endocardium of the left ventricle and extending up to the mitral leaflets.

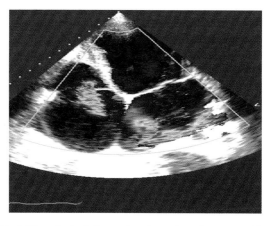

FIGURE 1.24. Apical four chamber view from a patient with endomyocardial fibrosis. Note the significant fibrosis that is involving the right ventricular apex (brightness) and the mitral regurgitation secondary to left-sided involvement.

Management of Mitral Regurgitation

Mild and moderate mitral regurgitation are well tolerated and do not require intervention apart from prophylactic antibiotics for potential infection. Severe mitral regurgitation which causes significant symptoms in spite of medical treatment warrants mitral valve surgery. Mitral valve repair is particularly satisfactory for posterior leaflet prolapse and occasionally for anterior leaflet prolapse. Timing of surgery is critical. While it should be at the earliest opportunity for papillary muscle rupture, it could be delayed for 1–2 weeks in case of chordal rupture until haemodynamics settle. This does not justify delaying intervention until patients develop irreversible left ventricular disease, indicated by an increase in end-systolic volume.

The treatment of papillary muscle dysfunction is that of left ventricular disease with particular aim at reducing left ventricular diastolic pressures. Mitral valve replacement in severe left ventricular disease should be avoided as it adds to the disruption of ventricular geometry and hence functional performance. Instead, an undersized mitral ring may be inserted to reduce the inflow diameter and hence the regurgitation, particularly in patients with dilated cardiomyopathy, whose ventricle is resistant to medical therapy.

Surgical Intervention for Mitral Regurgitation

Mitral valve prolapse, anterior and posterior leaflet, accounts for approximately 25% of overall mitral valve surgical procedures. A number of factors play an important role in predicting surgical outcome after correction of mitral regurgitation. Age-related operative mortality is in the order of 12% in patients above 75 years of age and 1% in younger patients [64]. Symptoms related to mitral regurgitation are also important predictors of outcome. While patients in NYHA class I and II carry a mortality of 0.5%

those in class III and IV have a surgical mortality of 5–10% [65]. Furthermore, the etiology of mitral regurgitation is another determinant of surgical outcome, with a 1–3% mortality in rheumatic mitral valve disease, compared to 9% in ischaemic mitral regurgitation [66]. In addition, the more complex the surgical procedure the higher the surgical risk. Finally, ventricular dysfunction adds to the surgical risk. There is a continuous relationship between left ventricular end-systolic measurements and the clinical outcome: a systolic volume of 50 mm/m^2 and an end-systolic dimension larger than 45–50 mm [67, 68] have been identified as the most sensitive parameters for selecting patients with ventricular dysfunction. Other risk factors include left atrial size, pulmonary hypertension, left ventricular end-diastolic pressure and reduced right ventricular systolic function, less than 50%.

Mitral Valve Replacement

Mitral valve replacement has a higher operative mortality (up to 30%) compared to aortic valve replacement for aortic stenosis, regurgitation or conservative operation for mitral stenosis. Although survival from mitral valve replacement surgery has improved significantly over the years, probably because of the better selection, improved myocardial preservation and surgical techniques, it remains of concern, particularly in patients with ischaemic mitral regurgitation; a 5-year survival is 75%.

Mitral homograft: The ideal valve would be a homograft in the mitral position. This can only be achieved by composing the mitral valve in a corded fashion and placing it attached to the annulus. This operation avoids cutting the papillary muscle heads and the chordae and preserves the continuity between the mitral valve apparatus and the left ventricle. Such attempts have proved uniformly unsuccessful. Pulmonary autograft has also been used in the mitral position (top-hat) with satisfactory results but in only a small group of patients in one or two centers. This procedure carries the advantage of the absent need for postoperative anti-coagulation as is the case with prosthetic mitral valves.

Mitral valve prosthesis: Mitral valve replacement by a mechanical or bioprosthesis is the only option for irreparable valves. It has a very satisfactory success rate, particularly when papillary muscles and chordae are preserved. Factors affecting valve choice are mainly the contraindication for anti-coagulants for mechanical valve. Bileaflet or tilting disc is currently the most commonly used mechanical valves.

Mitral Valve Repair

The concept behind mitral valve repair is to preserve the integrity of the mitral valve which results in a much better clinical outcome for patients with mitral regurgitation. Preservation of the chordal attachment is crucial in this operation which keeps the continuity between the mitral leaflets and the papillary muscle which controls the long axis function of the left ventricle. This also affects the sphericity of the left ventricle and hence the overall performance of the cavity. Mitral valve repair avoids the use of anti-coagulants that are needed for life in patients with mechanical prostheses. Even those who develop atrial fibrillation from mitral valve repair might not need the higher dose of anti-coagulants necessary for those who receive a mechanical valve. The most common procedure for mitral valve repair is the quadrilateral resection of the posterior leaflet, removing excess valve tissue, reapproximation of the scallops and annulus reduction with or without mitral annuloplasty. The success rate of this technique is in the order of 90%. Although historically anterior leaflet repair had been less easy than the posterior leaflet, recent advances have made it as successful as a posterior leaflet [63]. An alternative approach is by using the Alfieri repair which involves suturing the posterior and anterior leaflets together in the central section and creating a double orifice mitral valve. This approach is not widely accepted in the surgical community. In addition to mitral repair, patients with atrial fibrillation may be considered for arrhythmia ablation, by surgical or radiofrequency technique in order to restore sinus rhythm. Results of the combined procedure have been satisfactory with 80% of patients reverting to sinus rhythm, even with chronic atrial fibrillation before surgery. In primum interatrial communications and other forms of atrioventricular septal defect associated with left atrioventricular valve regurgitation, valve repair usually involves suturing the superior and inferior bridging leaflets together, within the left ventricle. Repair of the so-called isolated cleft of the anterior leaflet of the mitral valve can usually be performed by inserting a patch on the anterior leaflet to bridge the cleft. The results of this technique are generally excellent avoiding the need for mitral valve replacement in virtually every case.

Intraoperative Transesophageal Guidance

It is a routine practice now to use intraoperative transesophageal echocardiography that provides detailed perioperative assessment and detects early post-operative signs of valve dysfunction. Residual regurgitation can always be dealt with before closure of the chest and a second pump run can be established and the dysfunction corrected. A direct assessment of the mode of mitral valve repair can be provided which includes; direct leaflet repair, chordal replacement with Gore-Tex suture or annuloplasty through insertion of a mitral ring. Intraoperative transesophageal echo also helps in assessing left ventricular function before weaning off the bypass circulation. Finally, it identifies any entrapped air in the cardiac chambers. Of course, all these findings should be interpreted in the light of specific circumstances:

afterload effect, underloaded or overloaded ventricles, etc. In patients with combined left ventricular dysfunction in the setting of coronary artery disease and mitral regurgitation, intraoperative studies should identify the exact cause of early post-operative slow recovery whether it is ventricular dysfunction, valve regurgitation or possibly graft occlusion that needs direct visualization and correction. The same indications for transesophageal echo apply post-operatively in addition to the early collection of extra cardiac fluid that may have significant haemodynamic effects, irrespective of its volume [69, 70].

Follow-Up After Mitral Valve Surgery

The two main advantages related to surgical outcome for mitral valve repair over replacement are the lower mortality and deprivation of left ventricular systolic and diastolic dysfunction. Mitral valve repair has long term survival with maintained left ventricular function but the systolic function may fall if it was already low pre-operatively. The risk of endocarditis is much lower from mitral valve repair compared to replacement as is the thromboembolic risk. Patient selection is important for mitral valve repair. Although historical results of mitral valve repair for rheumatic regurgitation showed a success rate of 50%, better results have been recently reported with a re-operation in approximately 20% of patients at 10 years and in 40% at 20 years. Surgical repair for rheumatic mitral valve disease is also affected by rheumatic aortic and tricuspid valve disease. Current data suggest that even significant left ventricular dysfunction should not be used as an exclusion criterion for surgical correction of mitral regurgitation. The general belief is that a systolic dimension more than 50 mm indicates a poor prognosis and surgical intervention is unlikely to be of benefit. Pulmonary hypertension is another important predictor of outcome after mitral valve surgery which carries a poor prognosis. Correction of mitral regurgitation does not always guarantee normalization of pulmonary artery pressure, particularly if it was long-standing pre-operatively. This suggests that surgical intervention for mitral regurgitation should be considered before development of pulmonary hypertension.

Valve Replacement Complications

Although uncommon, a number of complications may potentially occur after mitral valve replacement which includes paraprosthetic leak and structural valve failure: calcification, tear of leaflet from valve perforation, obstructed prosthesis due to thrombosis or calcification, thromboembolism, endocarditis or conduction defects.

1) *Paraprosthetic regurgitation*: This may vary from mild to severe. In the presence of mechanical valves, color Doppler in the transthoracic echo cannot display a uniform regurgitant jet due to the mechanical reflection and therefore may underestimate its importance. A normalized left ventricular septal motion suggests significant leak. Transesophageal echo, however, is much more sensitive since the valve metal does not distract the ultrasound beam. Although it tends to overestimate the regurgitation, it can locate the exact site of the leak. Combining left ventricular activity on the M-mode and transesophageal color flow provides a fairly accurate means of assessment Figure 1.25.

2) *Disintegrating mitral bioprosthesis*: Although xenografts have their advantages over mechanical prostheses their expected durability is approximately 8 years, and they should thus be followed up annually. Once xenografts show signs of deterioration with rupture or tear of leaflets they should be replaced as soon as possible, regardless of the severity of regurgitation Figure 1.26.

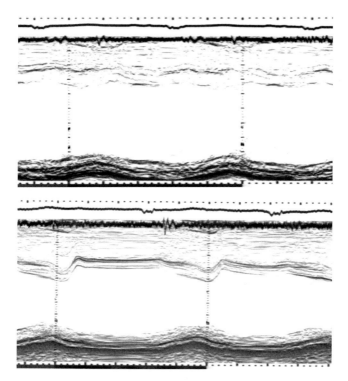

FIGURE 1.25. LV minor axis M-mode from a patient with St Jude mitral valve replacement. Note the normalized septal motion 12 months after surgery suggesting significant leak.

3) *Obstructed mitral prosthesis*: This is a very uncommon complication which is mainly due to thrombus formation on the valve that prevents its movement. Rapid development of pulmonary edema in a patient with mitral valve prosthesis suggests significant valve dysfunction with associated secondary pulmonary hypertension until otherwise proved. When confirmed an emergency valve replacement is the only management Figure 1.27.

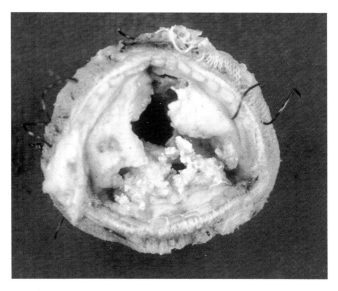

FIGURE 1.26. Pathological specimen from a disintegrated MV bio-prosthesis.

4) *Endocarditis*: Infection of a mitral valve prosthesis is not uncommon. It is usually difficult to treat medically. Transthoracic echo may or may not show evidence of vegetation. Transesophageal echo provides clearer images of the valves. However, it should not be allowed to overestimate findings. Resistant infection may be eradicated only by valve replacement and debris clearing (Figure 1.28) Figure 1.29.

5) *Fibrin strands/thrombi*: Fibrin strands are basically an echocardiographic finding and can be seen on mechanical valves but they constitute no real clinical harm. They should be differentiated from vegetations **Figure 1.30.**

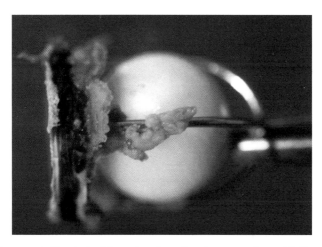

FIGURE 1.27. Apical four chamber view from a patient with Starr–Edwards valve in the mitral position. Note the high forward flow velocities giving rise to a mean pressure drop of 20 mmHg on CW Doppler.

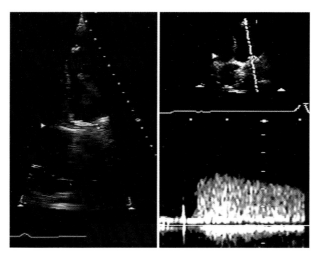

FIGURE 1.28. Starr–Edwards ball cage metallic valve excised from the mitral position. Note the stuck ball in the cage by the surrounding clot.

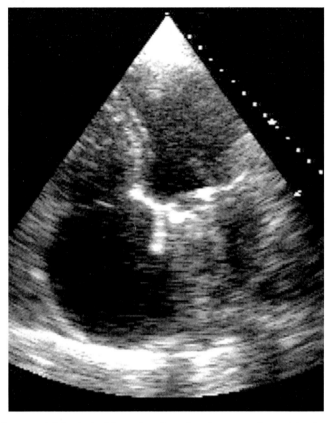

FIGURE 1.29. Apical four chamber view from a patient with mitral xenograft and large vegetation on the valve.

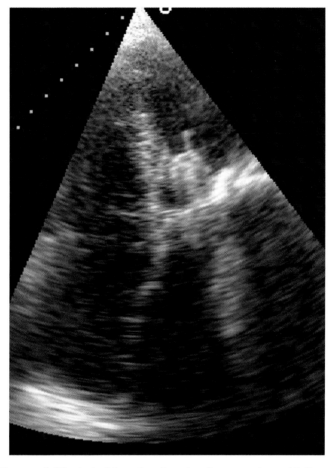

FIGURE 1.30. Apical four chamber view from a patient with Starr–Edwards mitral prosthesis with small fibrin strands attached to it.

References

1. National Center for Health Statistics: Vital and Health Statistics: Series 13, Hyattsville, MD. Centers for Disease Control and Prevention 1985–1999. 2006. Ref Type: Internet Communication.

2. Zhang W, Chung CS, Shmuylovich L, Kovacs SJ. Viewpoint: is left ventricular volume during diastasis the real equilibrium volume and what is its relationship to diastolic suction. J Appl Physiol 2007 Sep 27.

3. Kilner PJ, Henein MY, Gibson DG. Our tortuous heart in dynamic mode – an echocardiographic study of mitral flow and movement in exercising subjects. Heart Vessels 1997; 12(3): 103–110.

4. Henein M, Lindqvist P, Francis D, Morner S, Waldenstrom A, Kazzam E. Tissue Doppler analysis of age-dependency in diastolic ventricular behaviour and filling: a cross-sectional study of healthy hearts (the Umea General Population Heart Study). Eur Heart J 2002; 23(2):162–171.

5. Waller BF. Etiology of mitral stenosis and pure mitral regurgitation. In: Waller BF, editor. Pathology of the Heart and Great Vessels. New York: Churchill Livingstone, 1988; 101–148.

6. Moreyra AE, Wilson AC, Deac R, et al. Factors associated with atrial fibrillation in patients with mitral stenosis: a cardiac catheterization study. Am Heart J 1998; 135(1):138–145.

7. Alfonso F, Macaya C, Hernandez R, et al. Percutaneous mitral valvuloplasty with severe pulmonary artery hypertension. Am J Cardiol 1993; 72(3):325–330.

8. Wolf PA, Dawber TR, Thomas HE Jr., et al. Epidemiologic assessment of chronic atrial fibrillation and risk of stroke: the Framingham study. Neurology 1978; 28(10):973–977.

9. Hwang JJ, Li YH, Lin JM, et al. Left atrial appendage function determined by transesophageal echocardiography in patients with rheumatic mitral valve disease. Cardiology 1994; 85(2): 121–128.

10. Alpert JS. Mitral stenosis. In: Alpert JS, Dalen JE, Rahimtoola SH, editors. Valvular Heart Disease. Philadelphia: Lippincott Williams & Wilkins, 1999.

11. Smith MD, Handshoe R, Handshoe S, Kwan OL, DeMaria AN. Comparative accuracy of two-dimensional echocardiography and Doppler pressure half-time methods in assessing severity of

mitral stenosis in patients with and without prior commissurotomy. Circulation 1986; 73(1):100–107.

12. Kawahara T, Yamagishi M, Seo H, Mitani M, Nakatani S, Beppu S, et al. Application of Doppler color flow imaging to determine valve area in mitral stenosis. J Am Coll Cardiol 1991; 18(1):85–92.

13. Deng YB, Matsumoto M, Wang XF, Liu L, Takizawa S, Takekoshi N, et al. Estimation of mitral valve area in patients with mitral stenosis by the flow convergence region method: selection of aliasing velocity. J Am Coll Cardiol 1994; 24(3):683–689.

14. Nishimura RA, Rihal CS, Tajik AJ, Holmes DR, Jr. Accurate measurement of the transmitral gradient in patients with mitral stenosis: a simultaneous catheterization and Doppler echocardiographic study. J Am Coll Cardiol 1994; 24(1):152–158.

15. Hatle L, Angelsen B, Tromsdal A. Noninvasive assessment of atrioventricular pressure half-time by Doppler ultrasound. Circulation 1979; 60(5):1096–1104.

16. Hatle L, Angelsen BA. Doppler Ultrasound in Cardiology. 2nd ed. Philadelphia: Lea & Febiger, 1985.

17. Nakatani S, Masuyama T, Kodama K, Kitabatake A, Fujii K, Kamada T. Value and limitations of Doppler echocardiography in the quantification of stenotic mitral valve area: comparison of the pressure half-time and the continuity equation methods. Circulation 1988; 77(1):78–85.

18. Rothlisberger C, Essop MR, Skudicky D, et al. Results of percutaneous balloon mitral valvotomy in young adults. Am J Cardiol 1993; 72(1):73–77.

19. Horstkotte D, Niehues R, Strauer BE. Pathomorphological aspects, aetiology and natural history of acquired mitral valve stenosis. Eur Heart J 1991; 12(Suppl-B):55–60.

20. Sueda T, Imai K, Ishii O, et al. Efficacy of pulmonary vein isolation for the elimination of chronic atrial fibrillation in cardiac valvular surgery. Ann Thorac Surg 2001; 71(4):1189–1193.

21. Jatene MB, Marcial MB, Tarasoutchi F, et al. Influence of the maze procedure on the treatment of rheumatic atrial fibrillation – evaluation of rhythm control and clinical outcome in a comparative study. Eur J Cardiothorac Surg 2000; 7(2):117–124.

22. Abascal VM, Wilkins GT, O'Shea JP, Choong CY, Palacios IF, Thomas JD, et al. Prediction of successful outcome in 130 patients undergoing percutaneous balloon mitral valvotomy. Circulation 1990; 82(2):448–456.

23. Palacios IF, Block PC, Wilkins GT, Weyman AE. Follow-up of patients undergoing percutaneous mitral balloon valvotomy: analysis of factors determining restenosis. Circulation 1989; 79(3):573–579.

24. Wilkins GT, Weyman AE, Abascal VM, Block PC, Palacios IF. Percutaneous balloon dilatation of the mitral valve: an analysis of echocardiographic variables related to outcome and the mechanism of dilatation. Br Heart J 1988; 60(4):299–308.

25. Detter C, Fischlein T, Feldmeier C, et al. Mitral commissurotomy, a technique outdated? Long-term follow-up over a period of 35 years. Ann Thorac Surg 1999 Dec; 68(6):2112–2118.

26. Choudhary SK, Dhareshwar J, Govil A, Airan B, Kumar AS. Open mitral commissurotomy in the current era: indications, technique and results. Ann Thorac Surg 2003 Jan; 75(1):41–46.

27. Chauvaud S, Waldmann T, d'Attellis N, et al. Homograft replacement of the mitral valve in young recipients: mid-term results. Eur J Cardiothorac Surg 2003 April; 23(4):560–566.

28. Kumar AS, Choudhary SK, Mathur A, et al. Homograft mitral valve replacement: five years' results. J Thorac Cardivasc Surg 2000 September; 120(3):450–458.

29. Dahan M, Paillole C, Martin D, et al. Determinants of stroke volume response to exercise in patients with mitral stenosis: a Doppler echocardiographic study. J Am Coll Cardiol 1993; 21(2):384–389.

30. Sharma SK, Seckler J, Israel DH, et al. Clinical, angiographic and anatomic findings in acute severe ischemic mitral regurgitation. Am J Cardiol 1992; 70(3):277–280.

31. Lehmann KG, Francis CK, Sheehan FH, et al. Effect of thrombolysis on acute mitral regurgitation during evolving myocardial infarction: experience from the Thrombolysis in Myocardial Infarction (TIMI) Trial. J Am Coll Cardiol 1993; 22(3): 714–719.

32. Gula G, Yacoub MH. Surgical correction of complete rupture of the anterior papillary muscle. Ann Thorac Surg 1981; 32(1): 88–91.

33. Rankin JS, Hickey MS, Smith LR, et al. Current management of mitral valve incompetence associated with coronary artery disease. J Card Surg 1989; 4(1):25–42.

34. Kihara Y, Sasayama S, Miyazaki S, et al. Role of the left atrium in adaptation of the heart to chronic mitral regurgitation in conscious dogs. Circ Res 1988; 62(3):543–553.

35. Davison G, Greenland P. Predictors of left atrial thrombus in mitral valve disease. J Gen Intern Med 1991; 6(2):108–112.

36. Devereux RB, Kramer-Fox R, Shear MK, et al. Diagnosis and classification of severity of mitral valve prolapse: methodologic, biologic, and prognostic considerations. Am Heart J 1987; 113(5):1265–1280.

37. Devereux RB. Recent developments in the diagnosis and management of mitral valve prolapse. Curr Opin Cardiol 1995; 10(2):107–116.

38. Virmani R, Atkinson JB, Forman MB. The pathology of mitral valve prolapse. Herz 1988; 13(4):215–226.

39. Renteria VG, Ferrans VJ, Jones M, et al. Intracellular collagen fibrils in prolapsed ("floppy") human atrioventricular valves. Lab Invest 1976; 35(5):439–443.

40. Weiss AN, Mimbs JW, Ludbrook PA, et al. Echocardiographic detection of mitral valve prolapse: exclusion of false positive diagnosis and determination of inheritance. Circulation 1975; 52(6):1091–1096.

41. Duren DR, Becker AE, Dunning AJ. Long-term follow-up of idiopathic mitral valve prolapse in 300 patients: a prospective study. J Am Coll Cardiol 1988; 11(1):42–47.

42. Ling LH, Enriquez-Sarano M, Seward JB, et al. Clinical outcome of mitral regurgitation due to flail leaflet. N Engl J Med 1996; 335(19):1417–1423.

43. Ross J, Jr. Left ventricular function and the timing of surgical treatment in valvular heart disease. Ann Intern Med 1981; 94(4 Pt 1):498–504.

44. Grigioni F, Enriquez-Sarano M, Ling LH, et al. Sudden death in mitral regurgitation due to flail leaflet. J Am Coll Cardiol 1999; 34(7):2078–2085.

45. Devereux RB, Kramer-Fox R, Kligfield P. Mitral valve prolapse: causes, clinical manifestations, and management. Ann Intern Med 1989; 111(4):305–317.

46. Dajani AS, Taubert KA, Wilson W, et al. Prevention of bacterial endocarditis: recommendations by the American Heart Association. JAMA 1997; 77(22):1794–1801.

47. Suma H, Isomura T, Horii T, Nomuram, F. Septal anterior ventricular exclusion procedure for idiopathic dilated cardiomyopathy. Ann Thorac Surg 2006 October; 82(4):1344–1348

48. Breithardt OA, Sinha AM, Schwammenthal E, et al. Acute effects of cardiac resynchronization therapy on functional mitral

regurgitation in advanced systolic heart failure. J Am Coll Cardiol 2003; 41(5):765–770.

49. Lowes BD, Gill EA, Abraham WT, et al. Effects of carvedilol on left ventricular mass, chamber geometry, and mitral regurgitation in chronic heart failure. Am J Cardiol 1999; 83(8): 1201–1205.

50. Dujardin KS, Enriquez-Sarano M, Bailey KR, et al. Effect of losartan on degree of mitral regurgitation quantified by echocardiography. Am J Cardiol 2001; 87(5):570–576.

51. Castello R, Lenzen P, Aguirre F, Labovitz AJ. Quantitation of mitral regurgitation by transesophageal echocardiography with Doppler color flow mapping: correlation with cardiac catheterization. J Am Coll Cardiol 1992; 19(7):1516–1521.

52. Upton MT, Gibson DG. The study of left ventricular function from digitized echocardiograms. Prog Cardiovasc Dis 1978; 20(5):359–384.

53. Ishitoya H. Recovery of left ventricular function afte rmitral valve replacement for chronic mitral regurgitation: optimal timing of operation according to long-term recovery. J Cardiol 2000 July; 36(1):37–44.

54. Helmcke F, Nanda NC, Hsiung MC, Soto B, Adey CK, Goyal RG, et al. Color Doppler assessment of mitral regurgitation with orthogonal planes. Circulation 1987; 75(1):175–183.

55. Miyatake K, Izumi S, Okamoto M, Kinoshita N, Asonuma H, Nakagawa H, et al. Semiquantitative grading of severity of mitral regurgitation by real-time two-dimensional Doppler flow imaging technique. J Am Coll Cardiol 1986; 7(1):82–88.

56. Spain MG, Smith MD, Grayburn PA, Harlamert EA, DeMaria AN. Quantitative assessment of mitral regurgitation by Doppler color flow imaging: angiographic and hemodynamic correlations. J Am Coll Cardiol 1989; 13(3):585–590.

57. Eren M, Eksik A, Gorgulu S, Norgaz T, Dagdeviren B, Bolca O, et al. Determination of vena contracta and its value in evaluating severity of aortic regurgitation. J Heart Valve Dis 2002; 11(4):567–575.

58. Klein AL, Obarski TP, Stewart WJ, Casale PN, Pearce GL, Husbands K, et al. Transesophageal Doppler echocardiography of pulmonary venous flow: a new marker of mitral regurgitation severity. J Am Coll Cardiol 1991; 18(2):518–526.

59. Nishimura RA, Tajik AJ. Determination of left-sided pressure gradients by utilizing Doppler aortic and mitral regurgitant

signals: validation by simultaneous dual catheter and Doppler studies. J Am Coll Cardiol 1988; 11(2):317–321.

60. Ren JF, Kotler MN, DePace NL, Mintz GS, Kimbiris D, Kalman P, et al. Two-dimensional echocardiographic determination of left atrial emptying volume: a noninvasive index in quantifying the degree of nonrheumatic mitral regurgitation. J Am Coll Cardiol 1983; 2(4):729–736.

61. Bargiggia GS, Tronconi L, Sahn DJ, Recusani F, Raisaro A, De Servi S, et al. A new method for quantitation of mitral regurgitation based on color flow Doppler imaging of flow convergence proximal to regurgitant orifice. Circulation 1991; 84(4): 1481–1489.

62. Hochreiter C, Niles N, Devereux RB, et al. Mitral regurgitation: relationship of noninvasive descriptors of right and left ventricular performance to clinical and hemodynamic findings and to prognosis in medically and surgically treated patients. Circulation 1986; 73(5):900–912.

63. Smedira NG, Selman R, Cosgrove DM, et al. Repair of anterior leaflet prolapse: chordal transfer is superior to chordal shortening. J Thorac Cardiovasc Surg 1996; 112(2):287–291.

64. Enriquez-Sarano M, Tajik AJ, Schaff HV, et al. Echocardiographic prediction of survival after surgical correction of organic mitral regurgitation. Circulation 1994; 90(2):830–837.

65. Tribouilloy CM, Enriquez-Sarano M, Schaff HV, et al. Impact of preoperative symptoms on survival after surgical correction of organic mitral regurgitation: rationale for optimizing surgical indications. Circulation 1999; 99(3):400–405.

66. Hendren WG, Nemec JJ, Lytle BW, et al. Mitral valve repair for ischemic mitral insufficiency. Ann Thorac Surg 1991; 52(6):1246–1251.

67. Zile MR, Gaasch WH, Carroll JD, et al. Chronic mitral regurgitation: predictive value of preoperative echocardiographic indexes of left ventricular function and wall stress. J Am Coll Cardiol 1984; 3(2 Pt 1):235–242.

68. Bonow RO, Carabello BA, Chatterjee K, et al. ACC/AHA 2006 guidelines for the management of patients with valvular heart disease: a report of the American College of Cardiology/American Heart Association Task Force on Practice Guidelines (writing Committee to Revise the 1998 guidelines for the management of patients with valvular heart disease) developed in collaboration with the Society of Cardiovascular Anesthesiol-

ogists endorsed by the Society for Cardiovascular Angiography and Interventions and the Society of Thoracic Surgeons. J Am Coll Cardiol 2006; 48(3):e1–148.

69. Czer LS, Maurer G, Bolger AF, De Robertis M, Resser KJ, Kass RM, et al. Intraoperative evaluation of mitral regurgitation by Doppler color flow mapping. Circulation 1987; 76(3 Pt 2):III108–III116.

70. Reichert SL, Visser CA, Moulijn AC, Suttorp MJ, vd Brink RB, Koolen JJ, et al. Intraoperative transesophageal color-coded Doppler echocardiography for evaluation of residual regurgitation after mitral valve repair. J Thorac Cardiovasc Surg 1990; 100(5):756–761.

Chapter 2
Aortic Valve Disease

Michael Henein and Joseph Maalouf

The aortic valve is a passive valve made up of three leaflets which assume the shape of half moons (semi-lunar). Opposite to the mitral valve there is no true aortic fibrous annulus but a complex root made up of the aortic wall sinuses, left ventricular myocardium and interleaflet fibrous triangles. The ostia of the coronary arteries are located within the aortic sinuses. The sino-tubular junction is an important anatomic landmark for surgical procedures. It may be that the leaflets of the aortic valve are not passive as they are rich in different types of nerve endings. The function and role of these 'nerves' remain obscure.

Aortic Stenosis

Pathophysiology

Aortic stenosis is caused by congenital, rheumatic or senile disease. It may be at subvalvar, valvar or supra-valvar level, the commonest being the valvar stenosis. Subvalvar aortic stenosis is caused by a membrane (shelf) or hypertrophied upper septal segment bulging into the outflow tract. Subaortic membrane is a congenital anomaly that commonly progresses

M.Y. Henein (ed.), *Valvular Heart Disease in Clinical Practice*,
DOI 10.1007/978-1-84800-275-3_2,
© Springer-Verlag London Limited 2009

with age. Hypertrophy of the upper septum is an acquired syndrome that affects the elderly, particularly those with long-standing hypertension. Supra-valvar aortic stenosis is rare and is commonly part of William's syndrome. The commonest congenital valvar aortic disease is the bicuspid aortic valve which may remain completely silent for years, but as age advances the leaflets become thickened and calcified resulting in significant reduction in valve area and raised transvalvar velocities and pressure drop (gradient) across the valve, a sign of stenosis.

a) Determinants of Aortic Gradient

In addition to the anatomical narrowing of the aortic valve, left ventricular function plays an important role in determining the transvalvar velocities. Patients with mild valve narrowing and hyperactive ventricle (e.g., hyperdynamic circulation) may present with overestimated velocities across the valve. Likewise, those with severe aortic stenosis and poor left ventricular function may have underestimated velocities and pressure drop. Additional significant aortic regurgitation may itself overestimate the degree of valve stenosis because of the increased stroke volume. Timing of peak velocity across the valve is a good indicator of the degree of aortic stenosis. While in mild stenosis, velocities peak in early systole, in severe stenosis velocities peak in mid-systole, in parallel with the rise in aortic pressure. The maximum instantaneous velocity (m/s) across the aortic valve corresponds to the maximum instantaneous pressure drop (mmHg) according to the modified Bernoulli equation, $P = 4V^2$. The traditionally measured aortic pressure gradient during cardiac catheterization using a pull-back technique as the difference between peak left ventricular and aortic pressure is a less satisfactory measure because the two peaks do not occur simultaneously. A further problem with estimation of the aortic gradient by cardiac catheterization occurs because left ventricular pressure may not be uniform and so the measured pressure difference depends on the location of catheter tip in the ventricle, particularly in the presence of significant hypertrophy as in most cases of aortic stenosis. The difficulty increases since aortic pressure depends on its distance from the valve leaflets and the aortic wall as well as the pressure recovery process in the aortic root [1]. Such estimates of aortic pressure gradient using catheter technique should thus be regarded as semi-quantitative.

b) Aortic Velocity and Valve Area

Aortic stenosis can be quantified as valve area which can be calculated from the Doppler velocity data using the continuity equation based on the fact that the flow rate across the stenotic valve and the normal subvalvar area are equal [2]. Therefore the valve area is calculated based on the relative increase in blood velocity across the aortic valve with respect to the subvalvar region and subvalvar cross-sectional area. Thus, an increase in peak velocity across the aortic valve by five times that of subvalvar velocity with a pressure gradient of at least 35 mmHg is consistent with a five-times drop in aortic valve area and suggests severe aortic stenosis. The important application of this principle is in patients with a moderate aortic pressure drop because of low stroke volume as a result of impaired left ventriclar function. Stress echocardiography is a useful investigation in these circumstances. The enhanced myocardial inotropy increases the pressure generated by the ventricle and the stroke volume ejected. Increased aortic pressure drop above 70 mmHg with stress in such patients at the time of symptom development is consistent with significant aortic stenosis. Despite various attempts to determine the most sensitive marker of aortic stenosis valve gradient (pressure drop) remains the most appropriate measure in clinical practice [3]. Hemodynamics of aortic stenosis fundamentally differ from mitral stenosis. While mitral stenosis severity depends on the relative pressure gradient between the left atrium and left ventricular cavity in diastole, severity of aortic stenosis depends on the pressure actively generated by the left ventricle during systole.

c) Left Ventricular Response to Aortic Stenosis

With the increase in outflow tract resistance in aortic stenosis, left ventricular wall stress increases and hypertrophy develops. This compensatory mechanism preserves overall ventricular systolic function. Most patients develop concentric left ventricular hypertrophy and increased mass which regresses after removal of the stenosis. Left ventricular subendocardial ischemia may result from long-standing ventricular hypertrophy and outflow tract obstruction, and diastolic left ventricular function also become impaired, resulting in increased end-diastolic pressure and left atrial pressure. Patients with untreated aortic stenosis may present very late with left ventricular cavity dilatation, reduced ejection fraction and dyssynchrony. Most aortic stenosis patients who are allowed to reach this degree of ventricular dysfunction complain of progressive breathlessness and finally pulmonary edema.

d) Coronary Circulation in Aortic Stenosis

Even in the absence of significant coronary artery disease (atherosclerosis), the coronary circulation plays an important role in the pathophysiology and clinical presentation of aortic stenosis. Proximal coronary artery size is often increased, probably as a compensatory mechanism to the increased myocardial oxygen demand because of left ventricular hypertrophy but coronary flow reserve remains suboptimal. This limited coronary flow reserve is manifested in the subendocardium, which may become irreversibly damaged. The more severe the aortic stenosis, the more impaired the subendocardial function [4]. Furthermore, left ventricular relaxation is usually prolonged in left ventricular hypertrophy which itself further reduces coronary flow. The combination of hypertrophy-related altered coronary flow and increased myocardial work probably contributes to the angina-like symptoms known in aortic stenosis, even in the absence of epicardial coronary artery disease [5]. Regression of left

ventricular hypertrophy after aortic valve replacement improves coronary flow reserve [6].

Etiology of Aortic Stenosis

1) *Congenital cusp malformation*: A single commissure is
   seen in infants and young children whereas bicuspid or
   quadricuspid valves are usually discovered incidentally in
   young adults Figure 2.1. Bicuspid and quadricuspid aortic
   valves do not usually give rise to any significant hemodynamic abnormality before adulthood, as long as the pressure drop across the valve is not significant. The resulting turbulence at leaflet level, however, adds to the pre-
   disposition of these valves to further deformation, fibrosis,
   calcification and infective endocarditis [7, 8]. In a bicuspid
   aortic valve the commissures are commonly transverse in
   position and rarely vertical. Mild aortic regurgitation and
   dilatation of the ascending aorta frequently co-exist with
   a bicuspid valve [9]. In such patients with congenital aortic leaflet disease diagnosis of aortic coarctation should be
   excluded since it is a common association. This should easily be achieved by supra-sternal echocardiographic imaging introgation of abdominal aortic Doppler velocity or
   magnetic resonance imaging. In congenital aortic stenosis,
   leaflet movement is limited at the tips rather than at the
   base, and therefore relying on M-mode echocardiography
   alone may be misleading.

   In bicuspid aortic valve disease the morphology of the
   leaflets varies. The two leaflets may be of equal size or
   more commonly they are unequal Figure 2.2. The larger
   leaflet almost always has a shallow raphe in its middle
   part [7]. The large leaflets are mostly anterior in position
   and both coronary arteries arise from the sinus above it.
   Bicuspid aortic valves are not intrinsically stenotic unless
   the leaflets themselves are also dysplastic or there is additional superimposed pathological change Figure 2.3. The

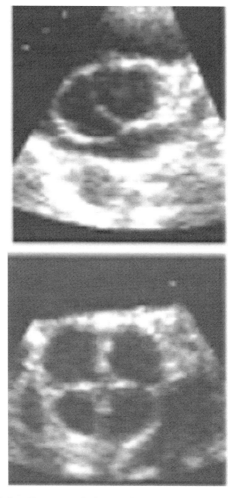

FIGURE 2.1.   Parasternal short axis view from two patients, one with bicuspid (*top*) and another with quadricuspid (*bottom*) aortic valve disease.

valves may become stenotic due to sclerosis and calcification or one of the leaflets may prolapse into the ventricle with subsequent development of valve regurgitation.

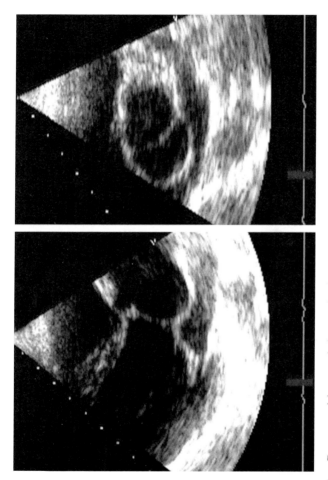

FIGURE 2.2.   Parasternal long and short axis views from a patient with bicuspid aortic valve showing eccentric closure point.

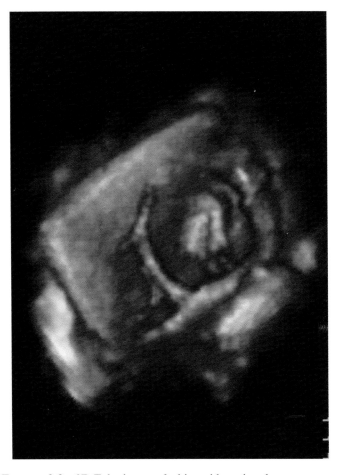

FIGURE 2.2.   3D Echo image of a bicuspid aortic valve.

Such congenitally deformed valves are highly susceptible to infective endocarditis.

2) *Congenital aortic tubular stenosis*: This is a rare congenital disease that presents with uniformly narrowed aortic root and proximal ascending aorta. Management of

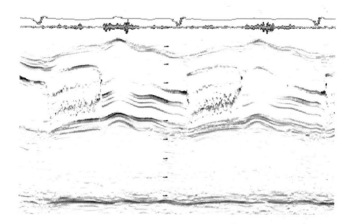

FIGURE 2.3. M-mode echogram from a patient with bicuspid aortic valve showing eccentric closure point, frequently seen in this condition. Note the fluttering leaflet as well.

this condition is complete resection and replacement of the aortic root and proximal (affected segment) ascending aorta. Aortic valve replacement alone in this condition does not correct the hemodynamic consequences of the narrowed left ventricular outflow tract.

3) *Subaortic stenosis*: This congenital lesion may be in the form of a fibrous membrane (ridge) below the aortic cusps or hypertrophied upper septum that bulges into the outflow tract. Subaortic membrane is a disease of the young that is usually in the shape of discrete, crescent-shaped fibrous shelf or membrane encircling the left ventricular outflow tract. It results in signs of ventricular hypertrophy and significant outflow tract gradient in the first three decades of life. Subaortic fixed narrowing is commonly associated with some degree of aortic regurgitation, probably caused by the disturbed vortices in the outflow tract and proximal ascending aorta [10, 11]. Other associated congenital cardiac conditions are atrial septal defect and coarctation of the aorta. When confirmed as the

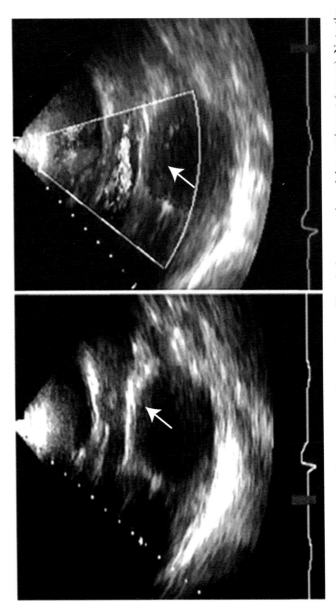

FIGURE 2.4.   Parasternal long axis view from a patient with tubular narrowing of the aortic root (arrow). Note the normal diameter of the ascending aorta distal to the site of narrowing.

cause of narrowing of the left ventricular outflow tract and symptoms, surgical excision of the subaortic membrane is the best line of treatment. Subaortic membrane lesion may recur years after surgery often due to incomplete resection at the initial operation and may be unpredictable Figures 2.5 and 2.6. Dynamic subaortic stenosis occurring early in life represents a component of hypertrophic cardiomyopathy. Muscular subaortic stenosis is more frequently seen in the elderly with a small left ventricular cavity irrespective of the cause of left ventricular hypertrophy [12]. When there is significant outflow tract narrowing it results in mid-systolic closure of the aortic valve. If the resting pressure drop (gradient) across the outflow tract is not significant in patients limited by exertional symptoms, exercise pharmacological stress is the ideal diagnostic tool

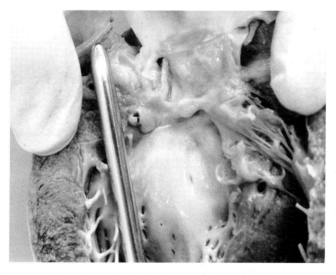

FIGURE 2.5.   A section in the long axis of the left ventricle and outflow tract from a patient with subaortic stenosis. Note the fibrous ridge beneath the aortic cusps.

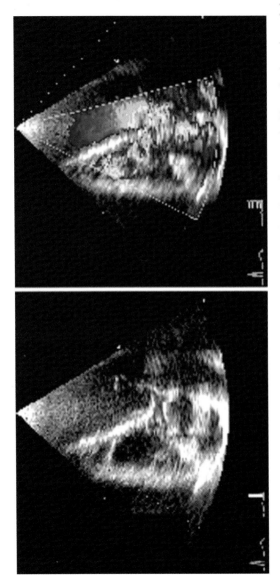

FIGURE 2.6.   (a) Apical five chamber view from a young patient with subaortic stenosis. Note the location of the membrane in relation to the valve cusps. (b) Color flow Doppler showing aliasing at the site of narrowing.

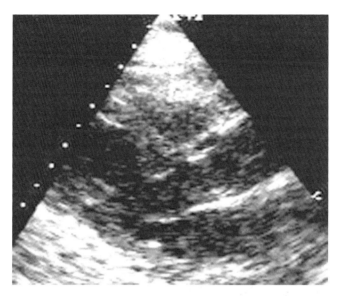

FIGURE 2.7.   Parasternal long axis view from an elderly lady with hypertrophied upper septum, bulging into the LV outflow. Note the normal aortic valve cusps.

for establishing the relationship between potential outflow tract obstruction and symptoms Figure 2.7.

4) *Supra-aortic stenosis*: This congenital anomaly is rare and is seen in association with William's syndrome [13–15]. It involves fibrous narrowing of the proximal segment of the ascending aorta distal to the coronary sinuses. Supra-aortic stenosis should be diagnosed early in life from routine 2D echocardiographic images with the color Doppler showing localized aliasing at the site of narrowing confirming the diagnosis. The severity of supra-aortic stenosis is quantified by continuous wave Doppler velocities Figure 2.8.

5) *Acquired aortic stenosis*:

   a) *Rheumatic aortic stenosis*: Rheumatic disease of the aortic valve is less common with that of the mitral valve

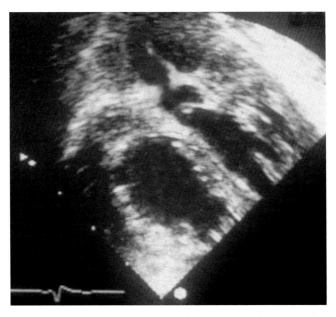

FIGURE 2.8. Parasternal long axis view from a patient with supra-aortic stenosis.

and is almost invariably associated with rheumatic mitral valve disease. Like mitral valve disease, rheumatic aortic leaflet involvement is associated with commissural fusion which can clearly be seen from short axis echocardiographic images of the aortic valve. As the disease progresses, the leaflets become fibrosed and calcified, resulting in valve stenosis. The degree of aortic stenosis is usually clinically underestimated when associated with significant mitral stenosis. Isolated rheumatic aortic stenosis is very rare Figures 2.9 and 2.10.

b) *Senile or degenerative aortic stenosis*: The commonest cause of aortic stenosis in the elderly is senile degeneration of the valve leaflets. It is caused by calcium

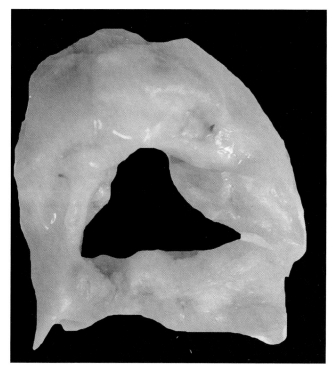

FIGURE 2.9. A picture of stenotic rheumatic aortic valve with fusion of the commissures, thickening and calcification of the leaflets.

deposition on the aortic surface of the valve [16]. As with the mitral valve, calcification in the elderly affects the base and slowly involves the body of the leaflets whereas with rheumatic disease the opposite occurs and the commissures fuse with calcification [17]. The calcium is deposited as large lumps within the body of each leaflet. Calcific aortic stenosis is an increasingly important disabling problem in an aging population, affecting 2% of people aged >65 years [16] Figures 2.11 and 2.12.

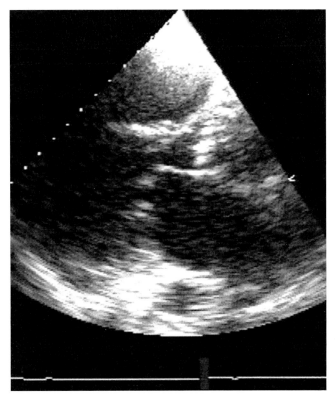

FIGURE 2.10.   Parasternal long axis view from a patient with combined rheumatic mitral and aortic valve disease.

Clinical Presentation

Symptoms: In patients with aortic valve disease, symptoms are mainly caused by the resulting ventricular disease.

Breathlessness: Mild aortic stenosis does not give any symptoms and even severe stenosis may be symptomatically silent. Breathlessness or exercise intolerance is the most common symptom in aortic stenosis. Long-standing hypertrophy and subendocardial ischemia may cause progressive deterioration

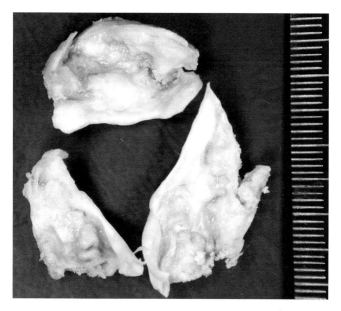

FIGURE 2.11. Pathology picture from an 80-year-old patient with senile degenerative calcification of the aortic valve. Note the nodular calcification in each leaflet.

of left ventricular function, raised end-diastolic pressure and left atrial pressure Figures 2.13, 2.14 and 2.15. The resulting raised pulmonary venous pressure causes breathlessness which initially appears on exertion then later at rest indicating severe additional left ventricular disease and pulmonary edema [18].

Chest pain: Angina-like symptoms are less common than breathlessness in aortic stenosis. The nature of chest pain is similar to that due to coronary artery disease but the underlying disturbed physiology is mismatch of oxygen supply and demand between the bulk of the myocardial mass and the coronary vascular bed, in the absence of epicardial coronary artery disease [19]. An additional factor to myocardial ischemia in aortic stenosis is the direct effect of abnormal

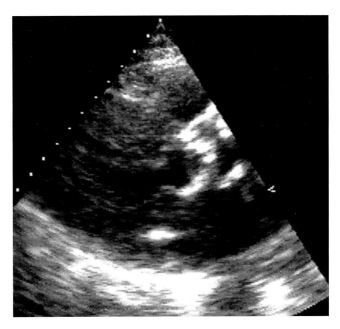

FIGURE 2.12. Parasternal long axis view from a patient with calcific AV disease. Note the extent of calcification on the leaflets and the root.

ventricular segmental relaxation on coronary flow in diastole as it raises the segmental wall tension and compromises subendocardial blood flow. This has been shown to be associated with significant broadening of QRS duration which normalizes after valve replacement as does segmental ventricular function [20].

Syncope: The third symptom in aortic stenosis is syncope which is due to either exertion-related hypotension as a result of the peripheral vasodilatation and the fixed resistance at the aortic valve level by stenosis, A-V conduction block by calcification, carotid sinus hypersensitivity or periods of ventricular arrhythmia or even fibrillation [21]. Similar

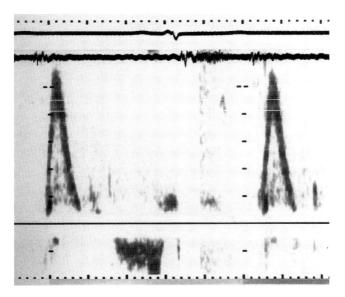

FIGURE 2.13.   Transmitral Doppler flow velocities from a patient with aortic stenosis limited by exertional breathlessness demonstrating restrictive filling pattern consistent with raised left atrial pressure.

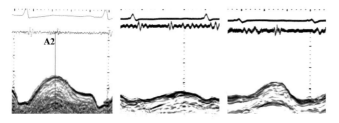

FIGURE 2.14.   Septal LV long axis recording from a normal (*left*) and a patient with significant aortic stenosis before (*middle*) and after valve replacement (*right*). Note the normalization of long axis lengthening velocities after surgery.

mechanisms underlie the commonly known sudden death in patients with aortic stenosis.

Physical examination: Carotid pulse examination is crucial in patients with aortic stenosis; its timing and amplitude

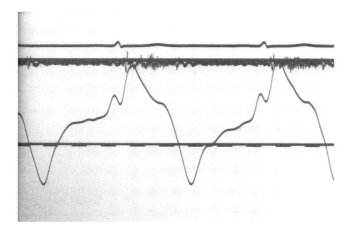

FIGURE 2.15.   An apexcardiogram showing raised end-diastolic pressure.

correlate closely with severity of stenosis [22]. A slowly rising low amplitude carotid pulse has high specificity for diagnosing severe aortic stenosis. Auscultation of the aortic area confirms long and harsh ejection systolic murmur. In most cases, the aortic stenotic murmur radiates to the carotids and the turbulent jet is directed superiorly into the ascending aorta. In a minority, the ejection systolic murmur may also be referred to the apex. Severe aortic stenosis is often associated with a systolic thrill over the aortic area. Significant additional aortic regurgitation might alter the nature and the timing of the aortic stenotic murmur. The second heart sound in aortic stenosis is typically single because of the limited cusp movement in heavily calcified valve. In young patients with severe aortic stenosis and mobile leaflets, the splitting of the second sound is reversed. A normal split second heart sound is a reliable sign for mild aortic stenosis. The third heart sound may be heard when left ventricular cavity dilatation and raised left atrial pressure have developed. A small Bernheim 'a' wave might appear in the jugular venous pulse associated with left atrial hypertrophy due to left ventricular hypertrophy.

Physiological echocardiographic studies with Doppler have disproved the old belief that Bernheim 'a' wave represents right ventricular inlet obstruction and confirmed it to be a sign of atrial cross-talk. The venous pressure remains normal (not raised) until late in the disease [23].

Investigations

Chest X-ray: The chest X-ray may be completely normal in patients with uncomplicated aortic stenosis. Post stenotic dilatation of the ascending aorta may be seen. Associated left ventricular disease leads to pulmonary venous congestion.

Electrocardiogram: Although most patients present with signs of left ventricular hypertrophy based on voltage criteria, some might present with a completely normal ECG. Advanced hypertrophy may be associated with non-specific T wave changes. With progressive left ventricular dysfunction QRS duration broadens and LBBB may develop. Inverted U wave may be seen in patients with severe left ventricular disease.

Echocardiography: Echocardiography is the investigation of choice for patients with aortic stenosis. It provides comprehensive information on the valve anatomy and function, left ventricular size and function, as well as any other associated disease that may contribute to patient's symptoms, e.g., mitral valve regurgitation. Transthoracic echocardiography is mandatory in all patients with aortic stenosis. Transesophageal echocardiography may assist in examining the aortic root and the proximal ascending aorta. The most clinically valuable measures of severity of aortic stenosis are transvalvular velocities mean gradient and value area. The blood flow sounds under 2D echocardiographic guidance assist in deciding on the optimum velocity recordings with the beam as parallel as possible to the jet direction. Peak velocities across the aortic valve are converted into a pressure drop (pressure gradient) using the modified Bernoulli equation P

$= 4V^2$. Color flow Doppler may determine the presence of mild aortic regurgitation in most patients with aortic stenosis. In those with impaired left ventricular function and raised end-diastolic pressure, Doppler recordings of aortic regurgitation should be carefully assessed to avoid overestimating the degree of regurgitation.

Assessment of Aortic Stenosis Severity

1) *Extent of leaflet separation*: An average value of aortic leaflet separation with respect to the aortic root diameter on an M-mode echo recording gives an idea about the severity of stenosis. The normal value is in the order of 70% of the aortic root diameter, mild stenosis 50% and moderate to severe stenosis <30% of the aortic root diameter. This method has its obvious limitations in overestimating the degree of valve stenosis in patients with severe leaflet calcification and those with significant left ventricular disease and low cardiac output [24–26].

2) *Continuous wave Doppler*: Peak pressure drop (gradient) across the aortic valve is calculated from the peak velocity recorded by continuous wave Doppler, using the modified Bernoulli equation $\Delta P=4V^2$, with a peak pressure of consistent with severe aortic stenosis Figure 2.16. Although this technique is the mainstay in assessing aortic valve instantaneous pressure drop it has its known limitations, particularly when compared with catheter measured transvalvar pressures. Continuous wave pressure drop values are often higher than the peak to peak (left ventricular-aortic) pressure obtained by the pull-back technique possibly because of the aortic site of the latter being often the velocity recovery area in the ascending aorta, thus underestimating the difference [27, 28]. Also, tip catheter placement in the hypertrophied ventricles commonly seen in this condition underestimates the real pressure drop across the valve. When comparing the mean aortic pressure, values of the two techniques are

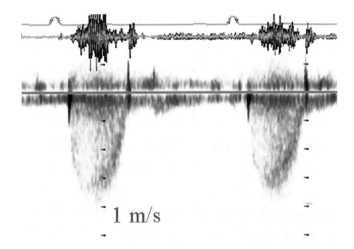

1 m/s

FIGURE 2.16. Continuous wave Doppler recording from a patient with severe aortic stenosis and a pressure drop of 70 mmHg. Note the systolic murmur on the phonocardiogram.

usually close, thus making the mean pressure better representative of the degree of valve stenosis with a mean pressure gradient of 40 mm Hg representing severe aortic stenosis in patient with manual LV systolic function and no significant aortic regurgitation. In addition, continuous wave Doppler velocities may underestimate aortic pressure drop if the ultrasound beam is not parallel to the high velocity jet (velocity varies inversely with cosine θ between the two) [29, 30]. Finally, in patients with severe left ventricular disease irrespective of its etiology, the modified Bernoulli equation may underestimate the degree of aortic stenosis because of the limited ability of the left ventricle to generate enough pressure to overcome the valve resistance Figures 2.17 and 2.18. Thus, more information on aortic value area can be obtained by using the continuity equation [31].

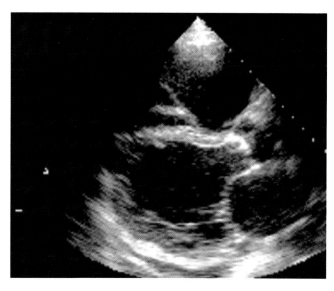

FIGURE 2.17. Parasternal long axis view from a patient with calcified aortic valve and dilated ventricle with poor systolic function.

3) *The continuity equation*: As discussed before the continuity equation is based on the principle of mass conservation and therefore it is the best method for assessing valve area. The blood volume passing through the subvalvular region, and consequently the ratio of blood flow velocities between aortic and subaortic areas, is inversely proportional to the ratio of the cross-sectional area. Subaortic area is calculated as $(diameter/2)^2 \times 3.14$. Aortic flow is measured from the velocity time integral calculated from the continuous wave Doppler and subaortic velocity integral from that of the pulsed wave Doppler velocity of the outflow tract. Aortic flow=aortic velocity time integral×area=subvalvar velocity time integral×area. Since ejection period is the same in the two areas, peak velocity may be used rather than its time integral. A velocity ratio <0.25 (subaortic) is 94%

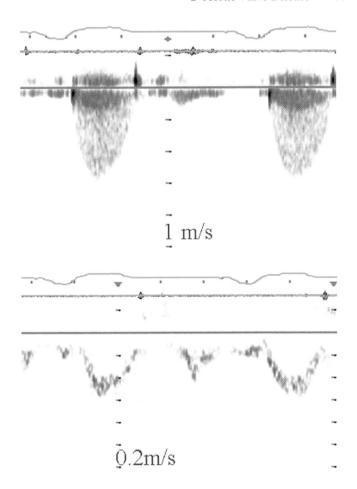

FIGURE 2.18.   Continuous wave Doppler from the same patient and pulsed wave Doppler velocities of the subaortic area. Note the >5 times increase in velocities between the two areas consistent with severe aortic stenosis.

sensitive in detecting severe aortic stenosis [32–35A]. A value area <0.7 cm^2 is consistent with severe stenosis. This method is ideal for assessing effective valve area in patients with poor ventricular systolic function and low-flow low-gradient state 35B].

Color flow Doppler: Although color flow Doppler displays the aortic flow jet beyond the valve, from which its narrow diameter could be measured, this technique is not routinely used for assessing aortic stenosis because of its limited reproducibility.

In addition to assessment of the valve anatomy and function in aortic stenosis, it is of great importance to assess left ventricular size and function, which assists in explaining patient's symptoms and in deciding on optimum timing for valve surgery, if needed. Echocardiography is unique in providing non-invasive accurate measurements of left ventricular dimensions and systolic function. This can easily be obtained by various techniques: M-mode dimensions at the base of the ventricle, Simpson's rule of cavity area 3D volume measurements. It also measures the degree of left ventricular hypertrophy and mass from which mass index can be calculated. Left ventricular mass and volumes can also be obtained using magnetic resonance imaging. Left ventricular Doppler filling pattern guides toward the assessment of left atrial pressure, particularly in patients limited by breathlessness. Most patients with aortic stenosis and left ventricular hypertrophy have a small early diastolic filling component and dominant late diastolic one. With progressive left ventricular disease and rise of end-diastolic pressure, the left atrial pressure increases and ventricular filling becomes of the restrictive pattern: Figure 2.19 a dominant early diastolic filling component with short deceleration time and a very small late diastolic filling component with flow reversal in the pulmonary veins. In such patients an apexcardiogram demonstrates the raised left ventricular end-diastolic pressure. Most patients presenting with this pattern of physiology have a dilated left atrium and even some may present

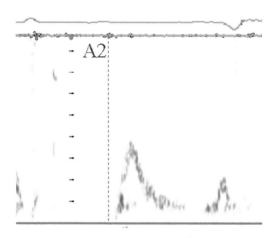

FIGURE 2.19. Apexcardiogram from a patient showing raised end-diastolic pressure and ventricular filling velocities showing restrictive physiology consistent with raised left atrial pressure.

with atrial arrhythmia. The extent of the commonly found mitral regurgitation can also be assessed by color and continuous wave Doppler. Left atrial pressure is reflected on the systolic right ventricular pressure which could be measured by continuous wave Doppler of the retrograde pressure drop across the tricuspid valve. An increased pressure drop across the tricuspid valve of more than 35 mmHg suggests some degree of pulmonary hypertension. As the right atrial pressure and size increase, the pressure difference between the right ventricle and right atrium underestimates the systolic pulmonary artery pressure. Absent normal inferior vena caval collapse and raised jugular venous pulse suggest a systemic venous pressure of 20 mmHg that should be added to the systolic pressure difference between the right ventricle and the right atrium. Mitral annular calcification is a very common finding in patients with severe aortic stenosis but it rarely contributes to any increase in atrial pressure or result in mitral stenosis.

5) *Stress echocardiography*: It has now become the investigation of choice, particularly in patients with moderate aortic stenosis, based on pressure gradient, who are limited by symptoms. With increase in heart rate, the increased blood flow across the valve differentiates between severe valve narrowing and severe left ventricular disease. A significant increase in transvalvular velocities and pressure gradient >70 mmHg or increase in mean gradient to over 30–40 mmHg reflects fixed valve area that does not increase and hence the diagnosis of severe aortic stenosis Figure 2.20. Failure of aortic velocities to increase significantly with stress suggests impaired left ventricular function as the cause of the low cardiac output and symptoms rather than aortic stenosis [36]. A valve area of <0.7 cm^2 that remains unchanged with stress is consistent with severe stenosis, particularly if there is evidence for adequate contractile reserve as evidenced by at least 50% increase in stroke volume [37].

6) *Cardiac catheterization*: High standard echocardiographic measurements of aortic stenosis severity are clinically very reliable and do not need to be reconfirmed by catheterization. Cardiac catheterization is needed only to assess possible additional coronary artery disease as a cause of unexplained ventricular dysfunction and also before aortic replacement surgery.

Natural History

Disease progression is generally slow in aortic stenosis. Symptoms are quite variable but overall reflect left ventricular disease. Patients with congenital bicuspid aortic valve tend to develop symptoms at an average age of 50 years compared to those with senile valve disease who develop symptoms at the age of 70–80 years. Patients with significant congenital aortic valve stenosis may develop symptoms earlier in life. Sudden

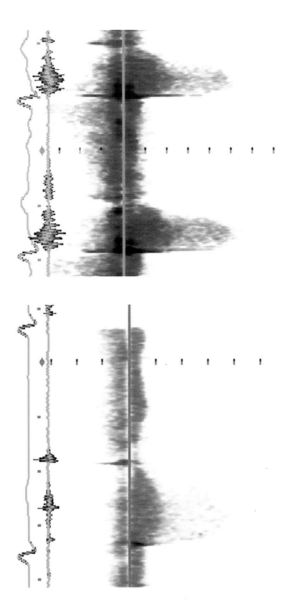

FIGURE 2.20. Continuous wave Doppler of transaortic valve velocities at rest (*left*) and peak stress (*right*) showing significant increase in velocities and consequently gradient from 55 to 120 mmHg and appearance of systolic murmur on the phonocardiogram.

death is a known outcome, 50% of patients with severe aortic stenosis who die have sudden death. Natriuretic peptides, despite being raised in severe aortic stenosis, do not provide any prognostic value. In contrast, raised aortic velocities and gradient and the rate of increase in velocities over time are the most accurate predictors of outcome in aortic stenosis [38]. The rate of deterioration of valve stenosis is faster in senile disease than rheumatic aortic stenosis. Once symptoms develop, the outcome is poor without surgical intervention, 5-year survival less than 50% [39]. Autopsy series showed that the average time from symptom development to death is 2 years in patients with exertional syncope, 3 years in those with dyspnea and 5 years in those with angina [40a]. It should be highlighted that prognosis is much better in patients with a high valve gradient rather than those with low gradient due to severe left ventricular disease. Recent data suggest that patients presenting with an ejection fraction <35% may fail to thrive even after successful aortic valve replacement surgery.

Approximately 50% of adults with aortic stenosis who need surgery have additional coronary artery disease. Patients with angina-like symptoms who have only mild aortic stenosis are likely to have significant epicardial coronary disease. However, a new onset of angina in patients with severe aortic stenosis may reflect a further deterioration of the degree of aortic stenosis and subendocardial ischemia. The difficult group of patients are those with moderate aortic stenosis and angina-like symptoms.

Treatment

Medical therapy: There is no medical therapy for aortic stenosis that may stop disease progression. Asymptomatic patients with mild or moderate aortic stenosis can be followed up, those with severe aortic stenosis need aortic valve replacement. A pressure gradient across the aortic valve of

>70 mmHg is a good indication for surgery, in symptomatic patients. Diuretics are important as well as B blockers as means for controlling the heart rate and its effect on symptoms and potential syncopal attacks. Once a patient develops raised left atrial pressure and pulmonary hypertension, the outcome even with surgery is less than satisfactory. Instructions on endocarditis prophylaxis and the use of antibiotics before dental and surgical procedures may be given [40b]. Patients with other co-morbidities and risks, in particular hyperlipidemia, should have their cholesterol and lipid levels well controlled. Recent studies have shown that patients who receive statins drop their rate of increase in valve calcification by 60% over 30-months follow-up as they reduce their LDL levels [41].

Surgical Treatment of Aortic Stenosis

The recent advances in the aortic valve surgery for aortic stenosis, in particular the procedure used, the improved method of myocardial preservation and earlier intervention, resulted in a significant fall in the surgical mortality to 3% in adults <70 years of age, in high volume centers. Older patients, particularly over the age of 80 years, with aortic stenosis tend to have a higher mortality. Concurrent coronary artery disease, ventricular dysfunction and pulmonary hypertension are important surgical risks [42, 43].

1) *Aortic valvuloplasty*: In contrast to mitral valvuloplasty, aortic valvuloplasty is only advisable in infants and young children in whom the valve leaflets are thin and pliable but in the majority a valve replacement is required at a later stage [44]. In the elderly, aortic valvuloplasty is not recommended in the management of stenotic valves. Open aortic valvotomy carries similar risks and benefits to valvuloplasty. The problem for the two procedures is the dysplastic valve leaflets for which 2D echo imaging provides

more detailed analysis on the extent of disturbed anatomy and leaflet behavior. If ever needed, aortic valvuloplasty may serve as a bridge to complete valve replacement in patients with ignored aortic stenosis who are in late stage heart failure [45].

2) *Aortic valve replacement*: Aortic valve replacement is the only recommended procedure in adults with severe aortic stenosis, particularly with calcified cusps. The outcome is complete relief of breathlessness, angina and syncope. Even in the presence of additional severe left ventricular disease, aortic valve replacement is the only choice, the results of which are very successful although the risk cannot be ignored. The lower the pre-operative ejection fraction, the higher the peri-operative mortality in these patients, thus optimal surgical timing is highly recommended [46–49]. Even in asymptomatic patients with severe aortic stenosis, the presence of left ventricular systolic dysfunction, concomitant significant coronary artery disease or pulmonary hypertension is an important indication for surgical intervention and valve replacement.

Mechanical or bioprosthetic valves: Over the years, technical improvement in the valve production has been remarkable with larger orifice area and greater resistance to thrombosis. Although the overall risk of mechanical valve implantation is low it increases with age, atrial fibrillation, hypercoagulable conditions and multiple valve replacement. Appropriate anti-coagulation therapy and close monitoring significantly reduce the risk. The commonest problem affecting less than 5% of patients with mechanical prostheses is a para-valvular dehiscence. While this may not always be hemodynamically significant, it may be responsible for a hemolytic anemia due to shear stress on red blood cells, and it is a focus for infective endocarditis. Valve dysfunction due to subvalvar tissue ingrowth, termed pannus, may interfere with valve opening and closure and cause reduction of the cross-sectional area. Mechanical and tissue valves are the commonest devices used for aortic valve replacement surgery. Their advantages and disadvantages are discussed in Chapter 6. Over the age of 65 years, there is an increasing trend to use a bioprosthetic valve as the durability has a mean of approximately 15 years and the bleeding complications of long-term anti-coagulation start to rise, reaching as high as 6%/year of patients by the age of 70 years [50–52]. There is increasing interest in the use of stentless valves in the aortic position, particularly in patients with additional severe left ventricular disease. The recovery of ventricular function in these patients has been shown to be much faster and complete when they receive stentless valves compared to stented valves [53–55]. Stentless porcine valves have been developed in order to increase availability. These valves are treated, in the same way as the stented valves, with glutaraldehyde. The durability of these valves at 8 years is 90%, which is at least 10% better than current stented porcine valves. Furthermore, stentless valves have been shown to have superior hemodynamics to stented valves early after operation and post-operatively to the second post-operative year. The difference has been demonstrated in its effect on early improvement of diastolic function and a fall in left ventricular mass to the normal range. They have also been shown to result in early recovery of function in patients with pre-operative poor left ventricular function Figure 2.21. It remains to be determined whether stentless valves are associated with increased long-term survival.

Homografts: The best option to replace a native valve is a human valve (homograft), but they are known for their limited availability. The ideal indication for aortic valve homograft replacement is in those with infective endocarditis that involves the aortic root and is associated with abscess formation. A mechanical valve replacement in this scenario limits the success of eradication of the infection. Aortic homograft implantation techniques have evolved from a two-layer subcoronary implantation to conduit implantation which involves replacing the valve and sinus of Valsalva by a full root and valve. This is still considered more

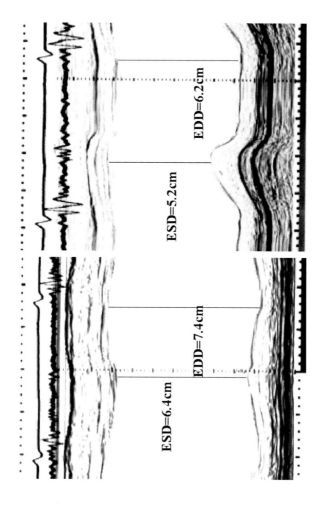

FIGURE 2.21. LV minor axis M-mode from a patient with severe aortic stenosis and poor LV systolic function (*left*) and 5 days after valve replacement with a stentless substitute (*right*). Note the significant fall in end systolic volume and recovery of posterior wall systolic function.

challenging compared with mechanical or tissue valve implantation. Under the age of 30 years, aortic homografts tend to fail within 10 years. In older patients, the mean survival of the valve is 15–18 years [56]. Long-term results of aortic homografts have proved encouraging with freedom from valve degeneration at 15 years in 75%. Both homografts and autografts once inserted have significantly lower incidence of endocarditis than any other valve because they contain no artificial material [57, 58]. However, they do degenerate eventually with calcification.

Pulmonary autograft or Ross operation: The Ross procedure goes back to 1967 [59] when Donald Ross transferred a patient's own pulmonary valve to the aortic position and inserted a homograft in the pulmonary position. This was a novel development because patients receive their own living valve in the aortic position. In children, these autograft valves, unlike any other valve substitute are capable of growth. They are also able to withstand high stress as seen during athletic exercise with heart rates above 170, where mechanical valves become increasingly inefficient [60, 61]. Aortic autograft surgery is more complicated and is usually reserved for specialist centers and for patients with a life expectancy in excess of 20 years. A pulmonary homograft is placed in the right ventricular outflow tract because of the lower pressures on the pulmonary circulation. Pulmonary valve homograft velocities tend to increase over the early post-operative months until it settles at a value of 2–3 m/s.

The Role of Echocardiography During Aortic Valve Surgery

Echocardiography has now become an essential imaging tool for intraoperative application in all valve surgeries. It has a vital role—before, during and soon after surgery [62, 63].

Pre-operative echocardiographic examination aims at

a) Assessing and quantifying the severity of aortic valve stenosis.
b) Assessment of the extent of left ventricular disease and maintaining its function.
c) Measuring aortic root diameter to guide the size of the valve substitute.
d) Measuring the pulmonary valve annulus when pulmonary autograft procedure is anticipated.
e) Assessing aortic root and ascending aorta diameter that may be included in the surgical procedure.
f) Identifying additional valve lesions whether as part of the same pathology or not.
g) It rules out the presence of a sizable Patent Foramen Ovale which could be dealt with at the time of surgery, particularly in patients with maintained left ventricular function.

Intraoperative echocardiographic study: Transesophageal echo at the beginning of surgery usually confirms transthoracic findings, although pressure drop estimation is difficult due to the technical limitation of aligning the continuous wave Doppler beam with the left ventricular outflow tract axis. Its additional value is mainly for excluding other lesions before operation, i.e., a small ventricular septal defect or other aortic shunts in patients with congenital valve disease or those with prior history of endocarditis. At the end of the operation, echocardiographic examination helps in confirming perfect placement of the valve substitute and in excluding any para-prosthetic regurgitation that can be dealt with before closing the chest. It also assesses the amount of entrapped air inside the ventricle during the de-airing stage. In patients with difficult weaning from the bypass machine echocardiography assesses the extent of ventricular loading. In patients with left or right ventricular disease due to compromised coronary filling, 2D imaging together with Doppler provide excellent means for assessing the extent of ventricular impairment and coronary velocities. Finally, echocardiographic examination assesses leaflet mobility, particularly in bileaflet mechanical valve prosthesis, rules out aortic hematoma or dissection, as well as significant tricuspid regurgitation as a result of intraoperative instrumentation.

Post-operative echo examination: Echocardiography is the investigation of choice for cardiac assessment in the early post-operative period. It provides a baseline finger print of the value substitute for future camparisons by measuring all function parameters including peak velocity, pressure gradient and valve area. It also allows established any patient-prosthesis mismatch. In patients with slow recovery, transthoracic or transesophageal echo provide detailed evaluation of the valve as well as ventricular function. Patients with high filling pressures may settle with vasodilators whereas those with under-filled ventricles require fluid loading. A high pressure pericardial collection irrespective of its volume may significantly contribute to the clinical deterioration in the early post-operative course. This should be drained in order to secure rapid recovery. Patients who develop high venous pressures within the first few days after surgery, who do not respond to diuretic therapy may have signs of post-operative tight pericardium, in the absence of pericardial effusion. A consistent increase in intrapericardial pressure leads to phasic (inspiratory) right heart filling and ejection which if ignored is followed by left heart (expiratory) phasic variations and pulsus paradoxus. This condition is benign and usually settles within days of the operation without a need for surgical intervention. Non-steroidal anti-inflammatory drugs may assist early recovery of this condition [63b].

Post-operative assessment and follow-up: In all surgical patients, early post-operative routine electrocardiographic, biochemistry, chest X-ray, echocardiographic and clinical assessment findings are very important to document. Valve function, velocities, the presence of aortic regurgitation, left ventricular size and function, right ventricular size and function and filling pressures represent very important data since they establish post-operative baseline against which patients follow-up would be measured. Ideally, all patients who have undergone aortic valve replacement should be followed up in specialized clinics and these may run by experienced nurses who are usually competent in applying strict protocols.

Left ventricular dysfunction: Most patients with good left ventricular systolic function before surgery remain with preserved systolic function post-operatively. In some, ejection fraction may increase post-operatively. Since it is difficult to predict recovery of poor ventricular function before surgery it is advisable to operate before the onset of ventricular dysfunction [64]. This highlights the need for more frequent pre-operative observations and assessment to detect early deterioration of ventricular function, even in the absence of severe stenosis. Although regression of left ventricular hypertrophy after surgery is expected intrinsic properties of the myocardium remain unchanged, due to fibrous deposition. Regression of interstitial fibrosis is known to be much slower than that of the myocardium [65]. This may have its implication on the persistent rise of end-diastolic pressure which makes patients limited by exertional breathlessness and hence underestimates the success of the aortic valve surgery. Finally, following aortic valve replacement and left ventricular mass regression a residual basal septal hypertrophy might remain. This may contribute to left ventricular outflow tract obstruction and dyspnea, particularly during exertion. These patients need heart rate control by a small dose of β blockers. Stress echocardiography provides confirmatory evidence for this dynamic outflow tract obstruction as a cause of patients′ symptoms at the time they drop their systolic blood pressure [66]. Patient prosthesis mismatch could be the mechanism behind slow/lack of recovery of ventricular function particularly in those with low gradient due to ventricular dysfunction [67].

Aortic valve replacement in the elderly: Age is not any more a contraindication to surgery. Aortic valve surgery is now provided to the elderly with a mean age of 80 years with great success, in large volume tertiary refinal centers which results in significant prolongation of life and improvement in the quality of life, particularly in those with no other significant co-morbidities. In a comparative study in the elderly, the outcome of those who received aortic valve replacement with a 10-year relative survival was 100% [68]. Surgical intervention in the octogenarians has also resulted in improvement of quality of life with a 5 years post-operative survival compared to only 1 year for the unoperated.

Percutaneous Aortic valve replacement: More recently, percutaneous aortic valve replacement has become a possibility. Results of this approach are becoming promising, particularly in experienced centers.

Aortic Regurgitation

Etiology

Aortic regurgitation is caused by either leaflet disease or aortic root dilatation.

1) *Rheumatic disease of the aortic valve*: It results in thickening of the cusps and fusion of the commissures with retraction of the leaflets and hence regurgitation **Figures 2.22** and 2.23.
2) *Aortic leaflet prolapse*: Aortic prolapse is a rare presentation that results from myxomatous degeneration of the aortic leaflets and consequently diastolic prolapse into the outflow tract of the left ventricle. This diagnosis can easily be made from echocardiographic images of the left ventricle and aortic root 'parasternal long axis view' as the

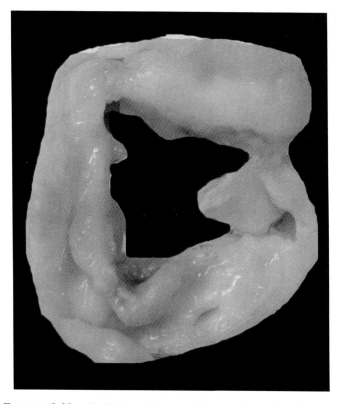

FIGURE 2.22.   Pathology picture of rheumatic aortic valve from a patient with severe aortic regurgitation showing leaflet thickening and retraction due to the extensive fibrosis.

leaflet tips meet below their aortic attachment level. Aortic prolapse may be associated with other conditions, e.g., mitral valve prolapse, bicuspid aortic valve disease or Marfan syndrome (MFS). Aortic prolapse may also represent a consequence of aortic valvuloplasty for valve stenosis in infants and children [69] Figure 2.24.

3) *Aortic valve infection (endocarditis)*: Infection of the aortic valve leaflets may be complicated by formation of vegetations on the surface of the leaflets which can break off

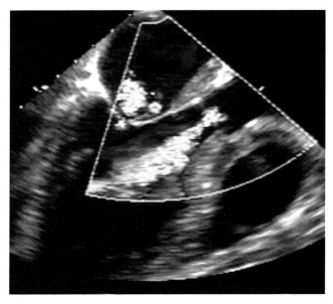

FIGURE 2.23.   Transesophageal echo from a young patient with combined rheumatic mitral and aortic valve disease demonstrating aortic regurgitation.

and embolize. The leaflets may also perforate. Valve infection complicated by vegetation may result in leaflet prolapse in diastole into the left ventricular outflow tract and hence aortic regurgitation. Aortic root abscess formation is associated with distortion of the valve leaflet and sinus morphology and is much more commonly associated with conduction disturbances [70]. Figures 2.25, 2.25 and 2.27

4) *Dilatation of the aortic root*: Aortic root dilatation is either seen in isolation or as part of the aneurysmal disease of the ascending aorta, commonly seen with MFS or isolated medial necrosis. Aneurysmal formation may rarely involve the coronary sinuses resulting in blood stagnation and aortic regurgitation. Aortic root dilatation may also be associated with more general connective tissue disease,

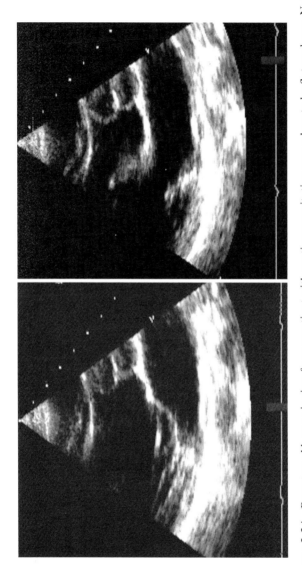

FIGURE 2.24. Parasternal long axis view from a patient with aortic regurgitation secondary to leaflet prolapse. Note the level of leaflet closure with respect to their attachment level to the aorta.

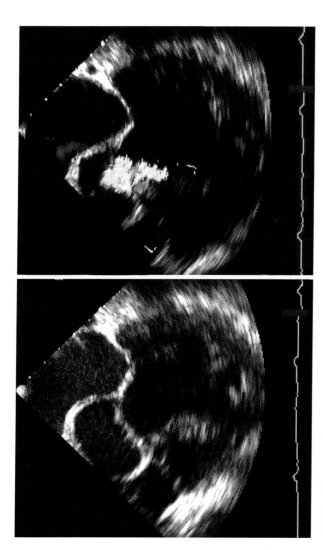

FIGURE 2.25.   TOE from a patient with severe aortic regurgitation secondary to bacterial endocarditis. Note the abscess cavity in the aortic root which changes its size and shape during the cardiac cycle.

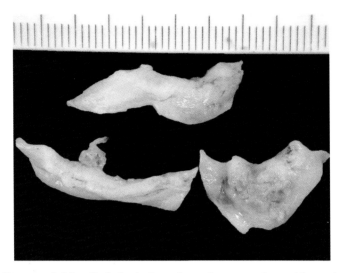

FIGURE 2.26.   Pathological specimen from a patient with aortic regurgitation secondary to infective endocarditis showing vegetation attached to the valve leaflet.

e.g., ankylosing spondylitis, rheumatoid arthritis, Reiter's syndrome or relapsing polychondritis. The increase in aortic root diameter reduces the area of apposition and hence poor leaflet coaptation and regurgitation Figures 2.28 and 2.29.

5) *Aortic dissection*: Aortic dissection is an uncommon pathology which can involve the aortic root or proximal ascending aorta. The cause of aortic regurgitation in the two conditions may differ. Dissection of the aortic root causes the flap to hold the leaflets opened in diastole, thus establishing direct access for blood from the aorta to the left ventricle. Aortic regurgitation caused by dissection of the ascending aorta results from disturbed normal blood vortices because of the high tension caused by the false lumen and the dissection flap Figures 2.30, 2.31 and 2.32.

6) *Ventricular septal defect*: Although a rare condition, a small subaortic ventricular septal defect may cause

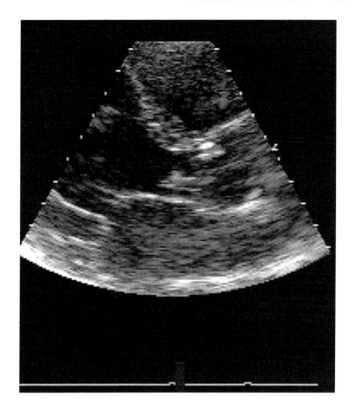

FIGURE 2.27. Parasternal long axis view from a patient with infected aortic valve showing a 2 cm long vegetation attached to the aortic cusp and moves freely in the aorta.

subaortic blood turbulence which results in spontaneously closed septal defect by a prolapsing aortic leaflet. This results in significant failure of competent leaflet coaptation and hence aortic regurgitation Figure 2.33.

7) *Syphylitic aortitis*: This is now a very rare cause for aortic regurgitation which results from aortic aneurysm and dilatation of valve area that may involve the coronary ostia.

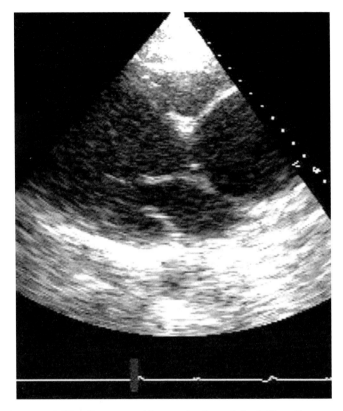

FIGURE 2.28.   Parasternal long axis view of the LV outflow tract and ascending aorta showing a fusiform aneurysm.

Pathophysiology

The left ventricular stroke volume in aortic regurgitation is significantly increased, which equals the forward stroke volume plus the regurgitant volume. The increased stroke volume is accommodated by an increase in left ventricular cavity size. This process is progressive in a similar fashion to that of mitral regurgitation though the degree of ventricular dilatation in aortic regurgitation is more than that with mitral

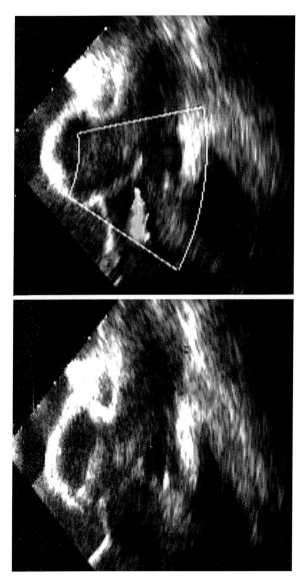

FIGURE 2.29. (a) Parasternal long axis view from a patient with aneurysmal aortic sinuses with a small clot in the right coronary sinus (cauliflower appearance). (b) Mild aortic regurgitation.

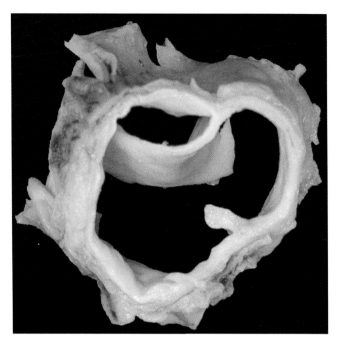

FIGURE 2.30.   Pathological section from a patient with dissection in the proximal ascending aorta forming a double barrelled aorta.

regurgitation. Another difference between the two conditions is the peripheral vascular resistance, which is significantly raised only in patients with aortic regurgitation. Therefore the combination of volume overload and raised peripheral resistance in aortic regurgitation results in a progressive increase in left ventricular wall thickness and mass. In uncomplicated aortic regurgitation, the left ventricular ejection fraction remains maintained, but as the disease progresses end systolic volume increases out of proportion to stroke volume. Eventually these changes lead to irreversible damage which persists even after surgical correction of the aortic regurgitation.

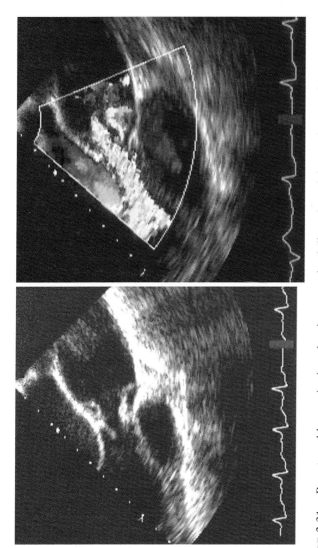

FIGURE 2.31. Parasternal long axis view showing a proximal dissection of the aortic root with the flap bouncing back into the left ventricle in diastole (*left*), holding the cusps opened and causing in aortic regurgitation (*right*).

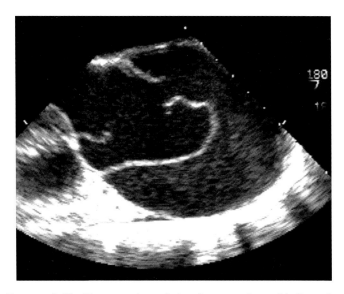

FIGURE 2.32. Transesophageal view from a patient with dissection of the ascending aorta 4 cm distal to the cusp level. Note the clotted false lumen.

Whether or not aortic regurgitation is accompanied by some degree of aortic stenosis due to intrinsic valve leaflet disease the increase in stroke volume causes high systolic velocities across the aortic valve. Pressure relations between the aorta and the left ventricle in diastole are of great importance, in particular the end diastolic pressure difference which depends not only on aortic but also on left ventricular end diastolic pressure. The higher the end diastolic pressure, the lower the pressure difference between the aorta and left ventricle. In mild aortic regurgitation, the pressure drop between the aorta and the left ventricle is maintained throughout diastole. With acute aortic regurgitation, the pressure difference between the aorta and the left ventricle falls to 15 mmHg or even less before end of diastole either because of the very low resistance at

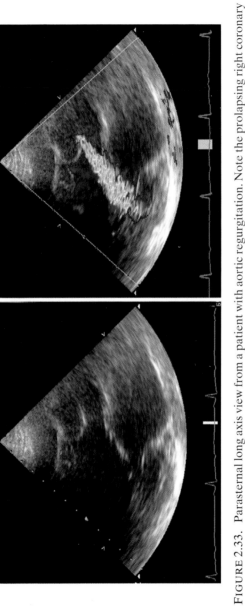

FIGURE 2.33. Parasternal long axis view from a patient with aortic regurgitation. Note the prolapsing right coronary cusp closing off a small subaortic VSD (*left*) and resulting in incompetent aortic valve (*right*).

the valve level or because the left ventricle is stiff, therefore a relatively small regurgitant volume causes a disproportionate left ventricular diastolic pressure rise. This disturbed physiology has major implications, since the reduced aortic-left ventricular diastolic pressure represents the pressure head supporting the coronary flow. Coronary autoregulation stops at a perfusion pressure difference between the aorta and the left ventricle of 40 mmHg. With acute aortic regurgitation or even severe chronic aortic regurgitation, the aortic-left ventricular pressure drop to 40 mmHg, result in significant myocardial ischemia and progressive ventricular dysfunction. While in chronic severe aortic regurgitation, this disturbed physiology may be tolerated in acute severe aortic regurgitation it may contribute to rapid clinical deterioration. In addition to the limitation of coronary flow by a raised ventricular end diastolic pressure it is affected by the increased oxygen demand of the myocardium as a result of the hyperdynamic ventricular state as well as the hypertrophy caused by the volume overload. This results in subendocardial ischemia, particularly with stress. In mild to moderate degrees of aortic regurgitation, isometric exercise and the fall in peripheral resistance increase ventricular systolic activity reduce and aortic regurgitant volume. With ventricular dysfunction, however, exercise causes further deterioration of ventricular systolic function and consequently the development of symptoms.

Acute aortic regurgitation results mainly from cusp perforation caused by infection or from an aging homograft or xenograft Figure 2.34. Although the left ventricular cavity becomes overloaded and active, overall ventricular function is maintained since it does not acutely dilate. Acute severe regurgitation results in early mitral valve closure (well before the onset of the QRS) Figure 2.35 and time restricted left ventricular filling [71]. Of course, this should be differentiated from early mitral valve closure associated with first degree heart block. The acute diastolic overload causes mid diastolic equalization of aortic and left ventricular pressures which has its effect on coronary circulation,

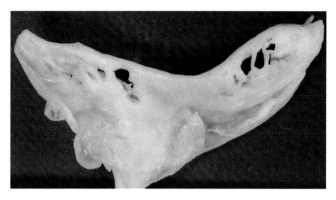

FIGURE 2.34. An infected aortic valve xenograft resulting in severe regurgitation due to a large hole in the right coronary cusp.

perpetuating rapid deterioration of ventricular function. Although the left ventricle may not be able to dilate acutely the large regurgitant volume will result in raised diastolic pressures with its subsequent additional effect on subendocardial blood flow and function. The acute rise in diastolic pressure can lead to a similar rise in left atrial and hence pulmonary venous and capillary pressures which in turn can result in pulmonary edema.

Clinical Presentation

Symptoms

Patients with aortic regurgitation may remain asymptomatic for a long time. The onset of symptoms, particularly breathlessness, coincides with the onset of left ventricular disease: a significant rise in end diastolic pressure and development of pulmonary venous hypertension. In the absence of coronary artery disease Angina is not a common symptom in aortic regurgitation but when it occurs, it should suggest significant subendocardial ischemia as a result of the mismatch between

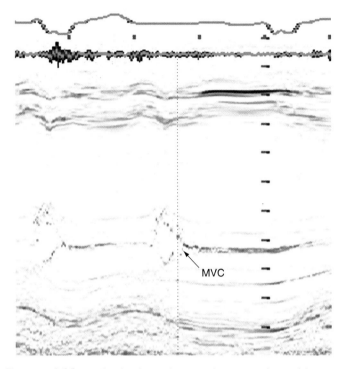

FIGURE 2.35.   Mitral valve echogram from a patient with acute aortic regurgitation showing early diastolic mitral valve closure.

the coronary artery flow and myocardial mass. Angina is more common in patients with acute rather than chronic aortic regurgitation. A sudden worsening of symptoms may reflect acute deterioration of the degree of aortic regurgitation or impairment of left ventricular function.

Physical Examination

The most important sign in severe aortic regurgitation is the collapsing pulse, due to the increased effective stroke volume in systole. Similar signs are shown in the carotid pulse which is usually bounding and left ventricular apex which is wide and displaced further into the axilla because of the left ventricular dilatation. Peripheral signs of aortic regurgitation are only seen in severe disease. These are all due to the large pulse pressure including the water hammer (Corrigan's pulse), systolic pulsations in the fingernail beds (Quinck's pulse) and the head movement with arterial pulsations. Flow reversal in the descending aorta is noted during the physical examination as systolic and diastolic bruits heard over the femoral arteries (Durozier's sign). Heart sounds do not demonstrate any specific change in aortic regurgitation. The classical murmur of aortic regurgitation is diastolic and of decrescendo nature which is loudest at the left sternal border. The murmur starts immediately after the second heart sound and continues throughout diastole. The murmur may be radiated to the right sternal border if it is caused by aortic root dilatation. The Austin–Flint murmur is a low pitched mid diastolic murmur that mimics that of mitral stenosis and is caused by the aortic regurgitant jet that limits the movement of the anterior leaflet of the mitral valve.

Physical signs in acute aortic regurgitation are quite different, based on the fact that the stroke volume does not increase by the same magnitude as in chronic regurgitation. The pulse pressure is normal or increased in patients who appear to have a low cardiac output, ventricular size is normal, peripheral signs are absent and the aortic regurgitant murmur is low pitched and mainly early diastolic. There may be a loud third heart sound. With development of left ventricular disease (increased end-systolic diameter >5.0 cm) and reduced effective filling period due to the raised end-diastolic pressure, a third heart sound and mitral regurgitation murmur may be heard.

Signs of aortic regurgitation may be modified with other accompanying conditions:

– In infective endocarditis and cusp perforation, the early diastolic murmur sounds musical in quality 'seagull murmur'. With homograft or xenograft degeneration, a loud systolic murmur may be heard and a classical prolapsing and thickened leaflet is seen on 2D echo images.

– In the presence of left ventricular disease or rheumatic mitral stenosis or pulmonary hypertension, the collapsing pulse and other signs of severe aortic regurgitation may be lost, although the early diastolic murmur remains.

– With very severe aortic regurgitation when the valve is virtually absent, the regurgitant murmur may be inaudible whereas the ventricular cavity is very active and the regurgitant jet diameter almost occupies the whole of the outflow tract.

Investigations

Electrocardiography: A 12-lead ECG may demonstrate increased voltage and a 'strain' pattern which correlate with the increase in left ventricular cavity dimensions, hypertrophy and wall stress. The voltage pattern may fall significantly after correction of the aortic regurgitation and regression of left ventricular mass [72]. Non-specific T wave changes may occur with exercise which either reflect the development of subendocardial ischemia or increase in systolic left ventricular volume. Increased QRS duration is a marker of left ventricular disease. Long PR interval may indicate aortic root abscess, particularly in those with clinical suspicion of endocarditis.

Chest X-ray: A chest X-ray may show increased cardiothoracic ratio and dilatation of the aortic root. This, on its own, can not be taken as a diagnostic investigation, particularly in the presence of echocardiography but is very useful for follow-up.

Echocardiography: Doppler echocardiography is an invaluable investigation for the assessment of aortic regurgitation patients. Two-dimensional images identify the exact cause of regurgitation. They show the valve anatomy: leaflet number, calcification or evidence for infection. The aortic root diameter and proximal ascending aorta can also be measured.

If this is not achievable on transthoracic images, transesophageal examination, particularly in patients with MFS or those presenting with dissection is always recommended. Finally, the left ventricular size, dimensions and ejection fraction can easily be measured as well as wall thickness and muscle mass calculated. Color Doppler detects the presence of aortic regurgitation and could be reliable for assessing its severity.

Assessment of Aortic Regurgitation Severity

a) *Active left ventricular cavity*: An increase in left ventricular end-diastolic volume and fall in end-systolic volume is compatible with a significant volume overload. The main difference between aortic and mitral regurgitation is that in the former ventricular loading occurs in early and mid diastole whereas with mitral regurgitation it is predominantly early diastolic. An increase in left ventricular minor axis end-systolic diameter >5.0 cm, or 2.5 cm m^2 in the presence of any overload suggests independent ventricular disease even in the absence of significant symptoms. At this stage, recovery of ventricular function even after complete correction of the valve incompetence can not be guaranteed [73a, 73b] **Figures 2.36 and 2.37.**

b) *Coarse fluttering of anterior mitral leaflet*: This is a common finding in aortic regurgitation. It is caused by the regurgitant jet interfering with the anterior leaflet opening in diastole. This sign, however, is not sensitive in estimating regurgitation severity [74] **Figure 2.38.**

c) *Color flow jet length*: Aortic regurgitation severity can roughly be assessed by measuring the distance of the regurgitant jet with respect to the valve level, either subvalvar (mild) or at mid ventricular cavity (moderate) or approaching the apex (severe). Although pulsed wave Doppler technique is sensitive and specific, it has always been used to offer only a semi-quantitative mean and therefore has become impractical for follow-up studies [75, 76]. This method is now hardly used.

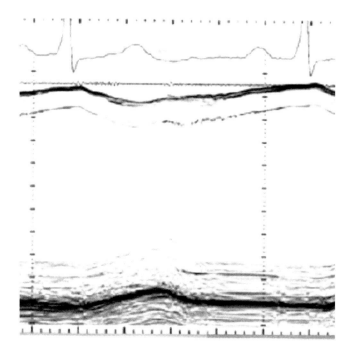

FIGURE 2.36.   LV M-mode recording from a patient with long-standing severe aortic regurgitation who developed left ventricular disease. Note the significant increase in ventricular end-systolic diameter and volume.

d) *Color flow jet diameter and area:* This is an accurate method for assessing regurgitation severity, particularly with native valves. A broad jet >12 mm that occupies >65% the aortic root diameter suggests severe regurgitation. Similarly, a color flow jet area that occupies over half that of the left ventricular cavity on the apical view (>7.5 cm^2) suggests severe regurgitation whereas an area of 1 cm^2 is compatible with trivial regurgitation. The major limitation of the latter is that the diameter and area, in particular, change over the course of diastole and may be affected by gain setting. Therefore for follow-up reasons a

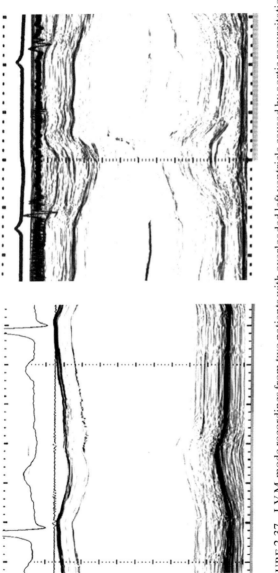

FIGURE 2.37. LV M-mode recordings from two patients with overloaded left ventricle caused by aortic regurgitation (*left*) and mitral regurgitation (*right*). Note the difference in loading pattern between the two: early and mid diastolic with aortic and mainly, early diastolic with mitral regurgitation.

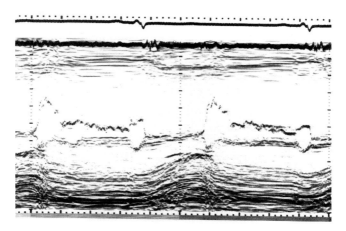

FIGURE 2.38. Mitral valve M-mode recording from a patient with aortic regurgitation. Note the course flutter of the anterior leaflet in diastole.

fixed time measurements should be considered (early diastole) [77] Figures 2.39 and 2.40.

e) *Continuous wave Doppler*: A rapid fall of aortic to left ventricular diastolic pressure by late diastole, particularly in the absence of raised LV end-diastolic pressure confirms severe regurgitation. A slow deceleration slope $<2m/s^2$ indicates mild regurgitation and a rapid slope $>4\ m/s^2$ indicates severe regurgitation. A pressure $\frac{1}{2}$ time of <300 ms also suggests severe regurgitation. Left ventricular end-diastolic pressure can be calculated as the late diastolic aortic-ventricular pressure drop deducted from the systemic diastolic blood pressure. In patients in whom the aortic regurgitation jet is directed toward the right ventricle, apical continuous wave recordings may be inappropriate, and the left parasternal window may be the optimal site [78–81]. In patients with left ventricular disease and raised end-diastolic pressure, aortic regurgitation pressure $\frac{1}{2}$ time should not be used since it overestimates the regurgitation severity Figure 2.41.

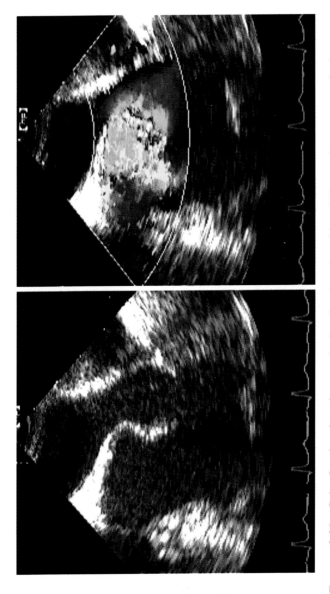

FIGURE 2.39. Color flow jet of aortic regurgitation showing a broad jet of 12 mm of severe regurgitation.

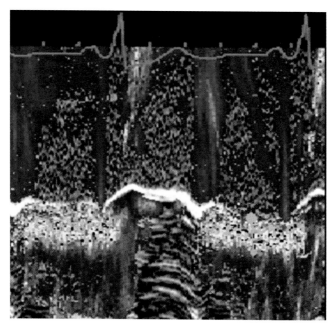

FIGURE 2.40. Color Doppler M-mode of the aortic root from two patients with mild and severe regurgitation. Note the difference in absolute and relative jet diameter with respect to the aortic root diameter.

f) *Diastolic flow reversal in the descending aorta or femoral artery* (Durozier's sign) confirms significant aortic regurgitation [82, 83] Figures 2.42 and 2.43.

g) *Continuity equation*: Aortic regurgitation severity is calculated as the relative regurgitant volume to the left ventricular stroke volume. Therefore the ideal way for estimating the regurgitant fraction is by measuring mitral valve area and diastolic velocity time integral and comparing it with that of the aortic valve. The difference is taken as the regurgitant fraction. The same method can be applied to measure the effective aortic regurgitant valve area. Velocity time integral at the valve level and valve area are compared with that 2 cm distal to the valve and valve

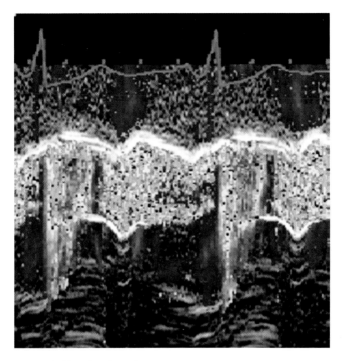

FIGURE 2.40. Continued.

regurgitant area is calculated. An area of 1.2 cm^2 suggests severe aortic regurgitation. Among the previous measurements of aortic regurgitation, severity of regurgitant area is considered the only load independent marker, however, is less reliable particularly with dilated aorta [84–87].

In patients with symptoms disproportionate to the degree of aortic regurgitation, diagnosis of left ventricular disease and raised filling pressures should be considered. In them, restrictive left ventricular filling may suggest potential additional pathology for ventricular disease rather than the aortic regurgitation itself, e.g. hypertension or coronary heart disease.

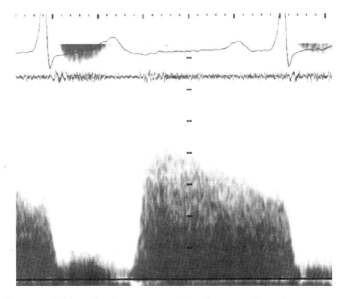

FIGURE 2.41. Continuous wave Doppler recording of severe aortic regurgitation. Note the fast deceleration and short pressure half time.

In acute aortic regurgitation echocardiography demonstrates clearly the cause of the disease: endocarditis with its complications or disintegrating homograft or bioprosthesis. M-mode echocardiography shows premature mitral valve closure which together with the left ventricular activity support the diagnosis of acute aortic regurgitation Figure 2.44.

Cardiac catheterization: The interest in using cardiac catheterization for assessing aortic regurgitation and its severity has declined by the fast development of echocardiography with its various modalities. Cardiac catheterization is only needed to confirm the presence of additional coronary artery disease, particularly before surgical intervention. Even this can now be acheived by multi detector CT angiography.

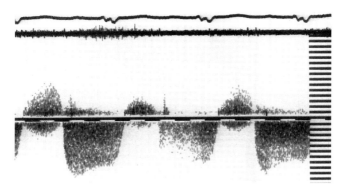

FIGURE 2.42.   Continuous wave Doppler from a patient with aortic regurgitation recorded from the left parasternal window demonstrating reversed signal.

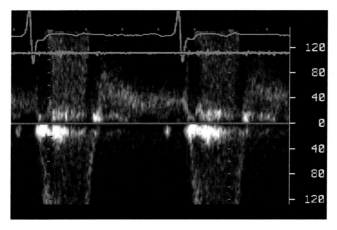

FIGURE 2.43.   Pulsed wave Doppler recording from the femoral artery from a patient with severe aortic regurgitation showing flow reversal in diastole.

Treatment

Medical treatment: Medical management of aortic regurgitation aims at slowing down its progression, supporting the

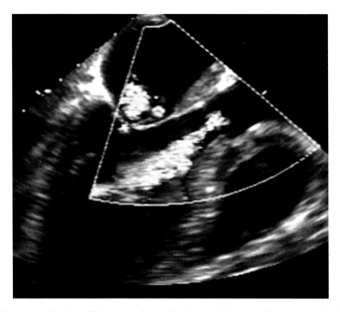

FIGURE 2.44.   Transesophageal echocardiogram from a patient
with aortic regurgitation on color flow Doppler.

left ventricle and determining the optimal time of surgical intervention. It is unlikely for mild aortic regurgitation
to progress rapidly to severe regurgitation and hence the
importance of the regular follow-up of such patients with
Doppler echocardiography. Identification of the exact etiology of aortic regurgitation should help in determining how
often patients should be followed up. Patients with mild
aortic regurgitation due to aortic root or ascending aorta
disease should be closely followed up compared to those
with stable valve disease. Patients with moderate or severe
aortic regurgitation may have no symptoms for years, as
symptoms, always reflect additional ventricular dysfunction.
Signs of left ventricular dysfunction are progressive increase
in end-systolic dimension/volume which should be considered as a serious indication for surgery even in the absence

of symptoms. Ejection fraction should not be taken as a marker of ventricular function in aortic regurgitation because of the volume overload and over estimation of the ejection performance. An end-systolic dimension up to 40 mm carries a good prognosis [88a, 88b], whereas a dimension more than 50 mm is associated with 20% probability of developing irreversible ventricular dysfunction, symptoms or even death over a course of 5 years. Other non-invasive investigations, e.g., CT scanning and cardiac magnetic resonance might play an important role in the follow-up of patients with aortic root or ascending aorta disease and 3D echocardiography for assessment of left ventricular size and function.

Aortic root: In the same way that patients with aortic regurgitation secondary to aortic valve disease are managed, those with aortic regurgitation caused by aortic root dilatation should be followed up with a view to assessing the aortic root dimensions and preventing its progressive dilatation and potential risk. An example of such patients is those with a bicuspid aortic valve who develop progressive dilatation of the aortic root because of the eccentric jet as well as the accompanying aortopathy [89]. Another group of patients that need regular follow-up and careful aortic root assessment are those with MFS. Aortic root aneurysmal dilatation and dissection are the major causes of morbidity and mortality [90]. β blockers are recommended for these patients because they decrease aortic wall stress, the blood pressure and the rate of pressure increase in systole [91]. Although MFS patients may remain completely asymptomatic the rate of aortic root dilatation is the most important risk factor [92]. While previous recommendations have suggested that aortic root or ascending aorta dimension larger than 55 mm is a good indication for surgical intervention [93], an earlier surgical intervention is now recommended, particularly in the presence of family history of dissection [94].

Afterload reduction: Medical treatment for the increased afterload in patients with aortic regurgitation is of significant importance in order to reduce the wall stress and the diastolic driving pressure across the valve. It decreases the pressure and the volume overload on the left ventricle and prevents progressive left ventricular dilatation and systolic dysfunction. This effect has been demonstrated [95] using angiotensin-converting enzyme inhibitors [96] and calcium-channel blockers [97]. The choice of the pharmacological agent for left ventricular afterload reduction depends on the other co-morbidities, e.g., coronary artery disease, kidney disease as well as patient tolerance.

Endocarditis prophylaxis: In line with prophylactic therapy, for all other valve diseases, for patients with aortic regurgitation oral hygiene should be encouraged and prophylactic antibiotics may be considered before dental, proctological, urological and gynecological surgeries [40b].

Management of Acute Aortic Regurgitation

Acute aortic regurgitation irrespective of its etiology should be managed as an emergency with surgical intervention. While diagnostic evaluation is in progress, the patient should be treated with afterload reduction. Aortic balloon counter pulsation is contraindicated in this condition because it increases the afterload. Those caused by infective endocarditis should receive optimum antibiotic therapy following blood culture and emergency valve replacement. It is always advisable that valve replacement for acute aortic regurgitation could be life saving.

Surgical Intervention for Chronic Aortic Regurgitation

Although patients with severe chronic aortic regurgitation may remain asymptomatic, surgical intervention should be offered, particularly when there is progressive increase in systolic ventricular dimension. A left ventricular end systolic dimension of 40 mm is a cut-off value for preserved left ventricular systolic function, particularly for an active ventricle. Predictors of outcome after valve surgery are severe aortic regurgitation, age, severe symptoms, exercise intolerance and evidence for left ventricular hypertrophy on echocardiography. Reduced by ejection fraction, increased end systolic dimension. Raised end diastolic pressure and the ratio of wall thickness to chamber dimension [98] have also been identified as potential predictor of outcome. An additional risk is the presence of coronary artery disease. These patients should be carefully evaluated by pre-operative cardiac catheterization or potentially multi-slice CT coronary angiography and receive myocardial revascularization surgery and coronary grafting at the same setting with aortic valve replacement surgery. There is evidence suggesting that patients with aortic regurgitation and ventricular dysfunction following successful valve replacement develop faster reverse remodeling and fall of left ventricular mass index if they receive a stentless rather than a stented valve [99]. Aortic valve replacement thus, should not be denied even if left ventricular systolic dysfunction is severe, olbeit the outcome including operaive mortality is worse than that in patients with good prognostic indicators.

Although surgical management of aortic regurgitation is based on conventional methods of valve replacement, as mentioned above in aortic stenosis, in recent years there has been a growing interest in conserving the native aortic valve. This has arisen partly because of the experience of aortic valve repair in acute and chronic Stanford type A dissection of the ascending aorta, and partly because in the western world, disease of the aortic root has become the commonest cause of aortic regurgitation [100].

Much recent interest has centered on the surgical management of MFS. Before the era of open-heart surgery, the majority of such patients died of rupture of the aorta often before the age of 30 years. In 1968, Bentall and DeBono described a composite graft–valve procedure in which a prosthetic valve was sewn into the proximal end of an artificial tubular graft, which in turn was anastomosed to the aortic annulus, with the coronary arteries grafted to the side of the tube [101]. This procedure completely removes the defective aortic segment most prone to dissection and rupture. After 30 years experience with this operation, a multi-center retrospective report demonstrated the very considerable success that has been achieved [102]. The 30-day mortality was 1.5% for 455 patients who underwent elective repair, 2.6% for the 117 patients who had an urgent repair and 11.7% for the 103 patients who required emergency repair. Because nearly half the patients with aortic dissection had an aortic root diameter of 6.5 cm or less at the time of operation it seems sensible to advocate prophylactic repair of aortic aneurysms in MFS's patients when the diameter of the aorta is well below that size.

Despite this, there are some disadvantages to the Bentall operation. These include all the known complications of mechanical prosthetic valves and the possibility of removing a potentially functional native aortic valve. Another option is a technique of radical excision of the aortic root and implantation of the coronary ostia (Fagan 1983). Like the Bentall operation, this achieves the objective of removing the defective aortic wall but in contrast, the patient's own valve leaflets are preserved, resulting in more normal valve function and the avoidance of the complications of an artificial valve. The long-term results of this procedure are excellent for elective operations [103]. Currently in experienced units, prophylactic operation is recommended when the aortic root or ascending aorta diameter, reaches 5.0 cm. Until that time, patients are generally kept under close scrutiny with a combination of echocardiography and MRA or spiral CT scans performed at 6 monthly intervals. In patients with a family history of a ruptured ascending aorta, elective surgery is recommended even if the diameter is less than 5 cm [104]. In all reported series, emergency repair of the ascending aorta invariably emerges as a strong predictor of early mortality. An alternative approach to surgical removal of the ascending aorta, for patients with strong family history of rupture is the aortic exostent. This procedure involves simulating the patient's own aortic root and ascending aorta using cardiac magnetic resonance 3D imaging programme followed by manufacturing a Dacron stent of similar size that is surgically inserted around the proximal part of the ascending aorta without a need for cardiopulmonary bypass circulation. Midterm results of the first series are quite satisfactory with no mortality or complications.

References

1. Levine RA, Cape EG, Yoganathan AP. Pressure recovery distal to stenoses: expanding clinical applications of engineering principles. J Am Coll Cardiol 1993; 21(4):1026–1028.
2. Zoghbi WA, Farmer KL, Soto JG, et al. Accurate noninvasive quantification of stenotic aortic valve area by Doppler echocardiography. Circulation 1986; 73(3):452–459.
3. Otto CM, Burwash IG, Legget ME, et al. Prospective study of asymptomatic valvular aortic stenosis: clinical, echocardiographic, and exercise predictors of outcome. Circulation 1997; 95(9):2262–2270.
4. Rajappan K, Rimoldi OE, Dutka DP, et al. Mechanisms of coronary microcirculatory dysfunction in patients with aortic stenosis and angiographically normal coronary arteries. Circulation 2002; 105(4):470–476.
5. Petropoulakis PN, Kyriakidis MK, Tentolouris CA, et al. Changes in phasic coronary blood flow velocity profile in relation to changes in hemodynamic parameters during stress in patients with aortic valve stenosis. Circulation 1995; 92(6):1437–1447.
6. Hildick-Smith DJ, Shapiro LM. Coronary flow reserve improves after aortic valve replacement for aortic stenosis: an adenosine transthoracic echocardiography study. J Am Coll Cardiol 2000; 36(6):1889–1896.
7. Beppu S, Suzuki S, Matsuda H, Ohmori F, Nagata S, Miyatake K. Rapidity of progression of aortic stenosis in patients with congenital bicuspid aortic valves. Am J Cardiol 1993; 71(4):322–327.
8. Pachulski RT, Chan KL. Progression of aortic valve dysfunction in 51 adult patients with congenital bicuspid aortic valve:

assessment and follow up by Doppler echocardiography. Br Heart J 1993; 69(3):237–240.

9. Hahn RT, Roman MJ, Mogtader AH, Devereux RB. Association of aortic dilation with regurgitant, stenotic and functionally normal bicuspid aortic valves. J Am Coll Cardiol 1992; 19(2):283–288.

10. Gewillig M, Daenen W, Dumoulin M, Van der HL. Rheologic genesis of discrete subvalvular aortic stenosis: a Doppler echocardiographic study. J Am Coll Cardiol 1992; 19(4): 818–824.

11. Borow KM, Glagov S. Discrete subvalvular aortic stenosis: is the presence of upstream complex blood flow disturbances an important pathogenic factor? J Am Coll Cardiol 1992; 19(4):825–827.

12. Henein MY, O'Sullivan C, Sutton GC, Gibson DG, Coats AJ. Stress-induced left ventricular outflow tract obstruction: a potential cause of dyspnea in the elderly. J Am Coll Cardiol 1997; 30(5):1301–1307.

13. Nasrallah AT, Nihill M. Supravalvular aortic stenosis: echocardiographic features. Br Heart J 1975; 37(6):662–667.

14. Usher BW, Goulden D, Murgo JP. Echocardiographic detection of supravalvular aortic stenosis. Circulation 1974; 49(6):1257–1259.

15. Weyman AE, Caldwell RL, Hurwitz RA, Girod DA, Dillon JC, Feigenbaum H, et al. Cross-sectional echocardiographic characterization of aortic obstruction. 1. Supravalvular aortic stenosis and aortic hypoplasia. Circulation 1978; 57(3): 491–497.

16. Lindroos M, Kupari M, Heikkila J, Tilvis R. Prevalence of aortic valve abnormalities in the elderly: an echocardiographic study of a random population sample. J Am Coll Cardiol 1993; 21(5):1220–1225.

17. Brandenburg RO, Jr., Tajik AJ, Edwards WD, Reeder GS, Shub C, Seward JB. Accuracy of 2-dimensional echocardiographic diagnosis of congenitally bicuspid aortic valve: echocardiographic-anatomic correlation in 115 patients. Am J Cardiol 1983; 51(9):1469–1473.

18. Panidis IP, Segal BL. Aortic valve disease in the elderly. In: Frankl WS, Brest AN, editors. Valvular Heart Disease: Comprehensive Evaluation and Management. Philadelphia, PA.: F.A. Davis, 1985; 289–311.

19. DePace NL, Nestico PF, Kotler MN, Mintz GS, Kimbiris D, Goel IP, et al. Comparison of echocardiography and angiography in determining the cause of severe aortic regurgitation. Br Heart J 1984; 51(1):36–45.

20. Collinson J, Flather M, Pepper JR, Gibson DG, Henein M. Reversal of ventricular dysfunction and subendocardial ischaemia following aortic valve replacement in patients with severe aortic stenosis. Circulation 2000; 102(18):11–661.

21. Imaizumi T, Orita Y, Koiwaya Y, Hirata T, Nakamura M. Utility of two-dimensional echocardiography in the differential diagnosis of the etiology of aortic regurgitation. Am Heart J 1982; 103(5):887–896.

22. Bonner AJ, Jr., Sacks HN, Tavel ME. Assessing the severity of aortic stenosis by phonocardiography and external carotid pulse recordings. Circulation 1973; 48(2):247–252.

23. Gibson DG. Valve disease. In: Weatherall DJ, editor. Oxford Textbook of Medicine. Oxford Medical Publications, 1996; 2451.

24. Chang S, Clements S, Chang J. Aortic stenosis: echocardiographic cusp separation and surgical description of aortic valve in 22 patients. Am J Cardiol 1977; 39(4):499–504.

25. Lesbre JP, Scheuble C, Kalisa A, Lalau JD, Andrejak MT. Echocardiography in the diagnosis of severe aortic valve stenosis in adults. Arch Mal Coeur Vaiss 1983; 76(1):1–12.

26. Williams DE, Sahn DJ, Friedman WF. Cross-sectional echocardiographic localization of sites of left ventricular outflow tract obstruction. Am J Cardiol 1976; 37(2): 250–255.

27. Berger M, Berdoff RL, Gallerstein PE, Goldberg E. Evaluation of aortic stenosis by continuous wave Doppler ultrasound. J Am Coll Cardiol 1984; 3(1):150–156.

28. Currie PJ, Seward JB, Chan KL, Fyfe DA, Hagler DJ, Mair DD, et al. Continuous wave Doppler determination of right ventricular pressure: a simultaneous Doppler-catheterization study in 127 patients. J Am Coll Cardiol 1985; 6(4):750–756.

29. Hatle L, Angelsen BA. Doppler Ultrasound in Cardiology. 2nd ed. Philadelphia: Lea & Febiger, 1985.

30. Lima CO, Sahn DJ, Valdes-Cruz LM, Allen HD, Goldberg SJ, Grenadier E, et al. Prediction of the severity of left ventricular outflow tract obstruction by quantitative two-

dimensional echocardiographic Doppler studies. Circulation 1983; 68(2):348–354.

31. Pellikka PA, Nishimura RA, Bailey KR, Tajik AJ. The natural history of adults with asymptomatic, hemodynamically significant aortic stenosis. J Am Coll Cardiol 1990; 15(5):1012–1017.

32. Kosturakis D, Allen HD, Goldberg SJ, Sahn DJ, Valdes-Cruz LM. Noninvasive quantification of stenotic semilunar valve areas by Doppler echocardiography. J Am Coll Cardiol 1984; 3(5):1256–1262.

33. Richards KL, Cannon SR, Miller JF, Crawford MH. Calculation of aortic valve area by Doppler echocardiography: a direct application of the continuity equation. Circulation 1986; 73(5):964–969.

34. Zoghbi WA, Farmer KL, Soto JG, Nelson JG, Quinones MA. Accurate noninvasive quantification of stenotic aortic valve area by Doppler echocardiography. Circulation 1986; 73(3):452–459.

35a. Oh JK, Taliercio CP, Holmes DR, Jr., Reeder GS, Bailey KR, Seward JB, et al. Prediction of the severity of aortic stenosis by Doppler aortic valve area determination: prospective Doppler-catheterization correlation in 100 patients. J Am Coll Cardiol 1988; 11(6):1227–1234.

35b. Bonow RO, Carabello BA, Kanu C, de Leon AC Jr, Faxon DP, Freed MD, Gaasch WH, Lytle BW, Nishimura RA, O'Gara PT, O'Rourke RA, Otto CM, Shah PM, Shanewise JS, Smith SC Jr, Jacobs AK, Adams CD, Anderson JL, Antman EM, Faxon DP, Fuster V, Halperin JL, Hiratzka LF, Hunt SA, Lytle BW, Nishimura R, Page RL, Riegel B. ACC/AHA 2006 guideliness for the management of patients with valvular heart diseases: a report of the American College of Cardiology/American Heart Association Task Force on Practise Guidelines (writing committee to revise the 1998 Guidelines for the Management of Patients With Valvular Heart Disease): developed in collaboration with the Society of Cardiovascular Anesthesiologists: endorsed by the Society for Cardiovascular Angiography and Interventions and the Society of Thoracic Surgeons. Circulation 2006; 114:e84–e231.

36. Monin JL, Monchi M, Gest V, et al. Aortic stenosis with severe left ventricular dysfunction and low transvalvular pressure gradients: risk stratification by low-dose dobutamine echocardiography. J Am Coll Cardiol 2001; 37(8):2101–2107.

37. Schwammenthal E, Vered Z, Moshkowitz Y, Rabinowitz B, Ziskind Z, Smolinski AK, et al. Dobutamine echocardiography in patients with aortic stenosis and left ventricular dysfunction: predicting outcome as a function of management strategy. Chest 2001; 119(6):1766–1777.

38. Rosenhek R, Binder T, Porenta G, et al. Predictors of outcome in severe, asymptomatic aortic stenosis. N Engl J Med 2000; 343(9):611–617.

39. Horstkotte D, Loogen F. The natural history of aortic valve stenosis. Eur Heart J 1988; 9(Suppl E):57–64.

40a. Frank S, Johnson A, Ross J, Jr. Natural history of valvular aortic stenosis. Br Heart J 1973; 35(1):41–46.

40b. Wilson W, Taubert KA, Gewitz M, Lockhart PB, Baddour LM, Levison M, Bolger A, Cabell CH, Takahashi M, Baltimore RS, Newburger JW, Strom BL, Tani LY, Gerber M, Bonow RO, Pallasch T, Shulman ST, Rowley AH, Burns JC, Ferrieri P, Gardner T, Goff D, Durack DT. American Heart Association Rheumatic Fever, Endocarditis, and Kawasaki Disease Committee; American Heart Association Council on Clinical Cardiology; American GHeaert Association Council on Cardiovascular Surgery and Anesthesia; Quality of Care and Outcomes Research Interdisciplinary Working Group. Circulation 2007; 116:1736–1754.

41. Pohle K, Maffert R, Ropers D, et al. Progression of aortic valve calcification: association with coronary atherosclerosis and cardiovascular risk factors. Circulation 2001; 104(16): 1927–1932.

42. Fremes SE, Goldman BS, Ivanov J, et al. Valvular surgery in the elderly. Circulation 1989; 80(3 Pt 1)177–190.

43. Malouf JF, Enriquez-Sarano M, Pellikka PA, et al. Severe pulmonary hypertension in patients with severe aortic valve stenosis: clinical profile and prognostic implications. J Am Coll Cardiol 2002; 40(4):789–795.

44. Buchwald AB, Meyer T, Scholz K, Schorn B, Unterberg C. Efficacy of balloon valvuloplasty in patients with critical aortic stenosis and cardiogenic shock – the role of shock duration. Clin Cardiol 2001; 24(3):214–218.

45. Blitz LR, Gorman M, Herrmann HC. Results of aortic valve replacement for aortic stenosis with relatively low transvalvular pressure gradients. Am J Cardiol 1998; 81(3): 358–362.

46. Connolly HM, Oh JK, Orszulak TA, Osborn SL, Roger VL, Hodge DO, et al. Aortic valve replacement for aortic stenosis with severe left ventricular dysfunction: prognostic indicators. Circulation 1997; 95(10):2395–2400.

47. Connolly HM, Oh JK, Schaff HV, Roger VL, Osborn SL, Hodge DO, et al. Severe aortic stenosis with low transvalvular gradient and severe left ventricular dysfunction:result of aortic valve replacement in 52 patients. Circulation 2000; 101(16):1940–1946.

48. Pereira JJ, Lauer MS, Bashir M, Afridi I, Blackstone EH, Stewart WJ, et al. Survival after aortic valve replacement for severe aortic stenosis with low transvalvular gradients and severe left ventricular dysfunction. J Am Coll Cardiol 2002; 39(8):1356–1363.

49. Hamamoto M, Bando K, Kobayashi J, Satoh T, Sasako Y, Niwaya K, et al. Durability and outcome of aortic valve replacement with mitral valve repair versus double valve replacement. Ann Thorac Surg 2003; 75(1):28–33.

50. John S, Ravikumar E, John CN, Bashi VV. 25-year experience with 456 combined mitral and aortic valve replacement for rheumatic heart disease. Ann Thorac Surg 2000; 69(4): 1167–1172.

51. Milano A, Guglielmi C, De Carlo M, Di Gregorio O, Borzoni G, Verunelli F, et al. Valve-related complications in elderly patients with biological and mechanical aortic valves. Ann Thorac Surg 1998; 66(6 Suppl):S82–S87.

52. Collinson J, Henein M, Flather M, Pepper JR, Gibson DG. Valve replacement for aortic stenosis in patients with poor left ventricular function: comparison of early changes with stented and stentless valves. Circulation 1999; 100(19 Suppl): II1–II5.

53. Jin XY, Zhang ZM, Gibson DG, Yacoub MH, Pepper JR. Effects of valve substitute on changes in left ventricular function and hypertrophy after aortic valve replacement. Ann Thorac Surg 1996; 62(3):683–690.

54. Jin XY, Pepper JR, Gibson DG, Yacoub MH. Early changes in the time course of myocardial contraction after correcting aortic regurgitation. Ann Thorac Surg 1999; 67(1): 139–145.

55. Rajappan K, Melina G, Bellenger NG, Amrani M, Khaghani A, Pennell DJ, et al. Evaluation of left ventricular function and mass after Medtronic Freestyle versus homograft aortic root

replacement using cardiovascular magnetic resonance. J Heart Valve Dis 2002; 11(1):60–65.

56. O'Brien MF, Harrocks S, Stafford EG, et al. The homograft aortic valve: a 29-year, 99.3% follow up of 1,022 valve replacements. J Heart Valve Dis 2001; 10(3):334–344.

57. Carr-White GS, Glennan S, Edwards S, Ferdinand FD, Desouza AC, Pepper JR, et al. Pulmonary autograft versus aortic homograft for rereplacement of the aortic valve: results from a subset of a prospective randomized trial. Circulation 1999; 100(19 Suppl):II103–II106.

58. Grocott-Mason RM, Lund O, Elwidaa H, Mazhar R, Chandrasakeran V, Mitchell AG, et al. Long-term results after aortic valve replacement in patients with congestive heart failure. Homografts vs prosthetic valves. Eur Heart J 2000; 21(20):1698–1707.

59. Ross DN. Replacement of aortic and mitral valves with a pulmonary autograft. Lancet 1967; 2(7523):956–958.

60. Oury JH, Doty DB, Oswalt JD, Knapp JF, Mackey SK, Duran CM. Cardiopulmonary response to maximal exercise in young athletes following the Ross procedure. Ann Thorac Surg 1998; 66(6 Suppl):S153–S154.

61. Porter GF, Skillington PD, Bjorksten AR, Morgan JG, Yapanis AG, Grigg LE. Exercise hemodynamic performance of the pulmonary autograft following the Ross procedure. J Heart Valve Dis 1999; 8(5):516–521.

62. Morocutti G, Gelsomino S, Spedicato L, Frassani R, Bernardi G, Da Col P, et al. Intraoperative transesophageal echo-Doppler evaluation of stentless aortic xenografts: incidence and significance of moderate gradients. Cardiovasc Surg 2002; 10(4):328–332.

63a. Sousa RC, Garcia-Fernandez MA, Moreno M, Tizon M, Valdeviesos M, Rubio M, et al. The contribution and usefulness of routine intraoperative transesophageal echocardiography in cardiac surgery. An analysis of 130 consecutive cases. Rev Port Cardiol 1995; 14(1):15–27.

63b. Oh JK, Hatle LK, Mulvagh SL, Tajik AJ. Transient constrictive pericarditis: diagnosis by two-dimensional Doppler echocardiography. Mayo Clin Proc 1993; 68:1158–1164.

64. Lund O, Nielsen TT, Pilegaard HK, et al. The influence of coronary artery disease and bypass grafting on early and late survival after valve replacement for aortic stenosis. J Thorac Cardiovasc Surg 1990; 100(3):327–337.

65. Lorell BH, Grossman W. Cardiac hypertrophy: the consequences for diastole. J Am Coll Cardiol 1987; 9(5):1189–1193.

66. Aurigemma G, Battista S, Orsinelli D, et al. Abnormal left ventricular intracavitary flow acceleration in patients undergoing aortic valve replacement for aortic stenosis: a marker for high postoperative morbidity and mortality. Circulation 1992; 86(3):926–936.

67. Monin JL, Monchi M, Kirsch ME, Petit-Eisenmann H, Baleynaud S, Chauvel C, Metz D, Adams C, Quere JP, Gueret P, Tribouilloy C. Low-gradient aortic stenosis: impact of prosthesis-patient mismatch on survival. Eur Heart J 2007 November; 28(21):2620–2626.

68. Kvidal P, Bergstrom R, Horte LG, et al. Observed and relative survival after aortic valve replacement. J Am Coll Cardiol 2000; 35(3):747–756.

69. Allen WM, Matloff JM, Fishbein MC. Myxoid degeneration of the aortic valve and isolated severe aortic regurgitation. Am J Cardiol 1985; 55(4):439–444.

70. Lau JK, Robles A, Cherian A, Ross DN. Surgical treatment of prosthetic endocarditis: aortic root replacement using a homograft. J Thorac Cardiovasc Surg 1984 May; 87(5): 712–716.

71. Botvinick EH, Schiller NB, Wickramasekaran R, Klausner SC, Gertz E. Echocardiographic demonstration of early mitral valve closure in severe aortic insufficiency: its clinical implications. Circulation 1975; 51(5):836–847.

72. Enriquez-Sarano M, Seward JB, Bailey KR, Tajik AJ. Effective regurgitant orifice area: a noninvasive Doppler development of an old hemodynamic concept. J Am Coll Cardiol 1994; 23(2):443–451.

73a. Henry WL, Bonow RO, Rosing DR, Epstein SE. Observations on the optimum time for operative intervention for aortic regurgitation. II. Serial echocardiographic evaluation of asymptomatic patients. Circulation 1980; 61(3):484–492.

73b. Chaliki HP, Mohty D, Avierinos JF, Scott CG, Schaff HV, Tajik AJ, Enriquez-Sarano M. Outcomes after aortic valve replacement in patients with severe aortic regurgitation and markedly reduced left ventricular function. Circulation 2002; 106:2687–2693.

74. Robertson WS, Stewart J, Armstrong WF, Dillon JC, Feigenbaum H. Reverse doming of the anterior mitral leaflet

with severe aortic regurgitation. J Am Coll Cardiol 1984; 3(2 Pt 1):431–436.

75. Esper RJ. Detection of mild aortic regurgitation by range-gated pulsed Doppler echocardiograhy. Am J Cardiol 1982; 50(5):1037–1043.

76. Ciobanu M, Abbasi AS, Allen M, Hermer A, Spellberg R. Pulsed Doppler echocardiography in the diagnosis and estimation of severity of aortic insufficiency. Am J Cardiol 1982; 49(2):339–343.

77. Tribouilloy C, Shen WF, Slama M, Rey JL, Dufosse H, Choquet D, et al. Assessment of severity of aortic regurgitation by M-mode colour Doppler flow imaging. Eur Heart J 1991; 12(3):352–356.

78. Beyer RW, Ramirez M, Josephson MA, Shah PM. Correlation of continuous-wave Doppler assessment of chronic aortic regurgitation with hemodynamics and angiography. Am J Cardiol 1987; 60(10):852–856.

79. Labovitz AJ, Ferrara RP, Kern MJ, Bryg RJ, Mrosek DG, Williams GA. Quantitative evaluation of aortic insufficiency by continuous wave Doppler echocardiography. J Am Coll Cardiol 1986; 8(6):1341–1347.

80. Masuyama T, Kodama K, Kitabatake A, Nanto S, Sato H, Uematsu M, et al. Noninvasive evaluation of aortic regurgitation by continuous-wave Doppler echocardiography. Circulation 1986; 73(3):460–466.

81. Masuyama T, Kitabatake A, Kodama K, Uematsu M, Nakatani S, Kamada T. Semiquantitative evaluation of aortic regurgitation by Doppler echocardiography: effects of associated mitral stenosis. Am Heart J 1989; 117(1):133–139.

82. Hoffmann A, Pfisterer M, Stulz P, Schmitt HE, Burkart F, Burckhardt D. Non-invasive grading of aortic regurgitation by Doppler ultrasonography. Br Heart J 1986; 55(3): 283–285.

83. Quinones MA, Young JB, Waggoner AD, Ostojic MC, Ribeiro LG, Miller RR. Assessment of pulsed Doppler echocardiography in detection and quantification of aortic and mitral regurgitation. Br Heart J 1980; 44(6):612–620.

84. Enriquez-Sarano M, Seward JB, Bailey KR, Tajik AJ. Effective regurgitant orifice area: a non-invasive Doppler development of an old hemodynamic concent. J Am Coll Cardiol 1994; 23(2):443–451.

85. Kitabatake A, Ito H, Inoue M, Tanouchi J, Ishihara K, Morita T, et al. A new approach to noninvasive evaluation of aortic regurgitant fraction by two-dimensional Doppler echocardiography. Circulation 1985; 72(3):523–529.

86. Reimold SC, Ganz P, Bittl JA, Thomas JD, Thoreau D, Plappert TJ, et al. Effective aortic regurgitant orifice area: description of a method based on the conservation of mass. J Am Coll Cardiol 1991; 18(3):761–768.

87. Zhang Y, Nitter-Hauge S, Ihlen H, Rootwelt K, Myhre E. Measurement of aortic regurgitation by Doppler echocardiography. Br Heart J 1986; 55(1):32–38.

88a. Borer JS, Hochreiter C, Herrold EM, et al. Prediction of indications for valve replacement among asymptomatic or minimally symptomatic patients with chronic aortic regurgitation and normal left ventricular performance. Circulation 1998; 97(6):525–534.

88b. Dujardin KS, Enriquez-Sarano M, Schaff HV, Bailey Kr, Seward Jb, Tajik AJ. Mortality and morbidity of aortic reguagitation in clinical practice: a long-term follow-up study. Circulation 1999; 99:1851–1857.

89. Edwards WD, Leaf DS, Edwards JE. Dissecting aortic aneurysm associated with congenital bicuspid aortic valve. Circulation 1978; 57(5):1022–1025.

90. Marsalese DL, Moodie DS, Vacante M, et al. Marfan's syndrome: natural history and long-term follow-up of cardiovascular involvement. J Am Coll Cardiol 1989; 14(2):422–428.

91. Shores J, Berger KR, Murphy EA, et al. Progression of aortic dilatation and the benefit of long-term beta-adrenergic blockade in Marfan's syndrome. N Engl J Med 1994; 330(19): 1335–1341.

92. Roman MJ, Rosen SE, Kramer-Fox R, et al. Prognostic significance of the pattern of aortic root dilation in the Marfan syndrome. J Am Coll Cardiol 1993; 22(5):1470–1476.

93. Gott VL, Pyeritz RE, Cameron DE, et al. Composite graft repair of Marfan aneurysm of the ascending aorta: results in 100 patients. Ann Thorac Surg 1991; 52(1):38–44.

94. Treasure T. Elective replacement of the aortic root in Marfan's syndrome. Br Heart J 1993; 69(2):101–103.

95. Bolen JL, Alderman EL. Hemodynamic consequences of afterload reduction in patients with chronic aortic regurgitation. Circulation 1976; 53(5):879–883.

96. Lin M, Chiang HT, Lin SL, et al. Vasodilator therapy in chronic asymptomatic aortic regurgitation: enalapril versus hydralazine therapy. J Am Coll Cardiol 1994; 24(4): 1046–1053.

97. Scognamiglio R, Rahimtoola SH, Fasoli G, et al. Nifedipine in asymptomatic patients with severe aortic regurgitation and normal left ventricular function. N Engl J Med 1994; 331(11):689–694.

98. Gaasch WH, Carroll JD, Levine HJ, et al. Chronic aortic regurgitation: prognostic value of left ventricular end-systolic dimension and end-diastolic radius/thickness ratio. J Am Coll Cardiol 1983; 1(3):775–782.

99. Collinson J, Flather M, Pepper JR, Henein M. Effects of valve replacement on left ventricular function in patients with aortic regurgitation and severe ventricular disease. J Heart Valve Dis 2004 Sep; 13(5):722–728.

100. Gott VL, Greene PS, Alejo DE, Cameron DE, Naftel DC, Miller DC, et al. Replacement of the aortic root in patients with Marfan's syndrome. N Engl J Med 1999; 340(17): 1307–1313.

101. Bentall H, De Bono A. A technique for complete replacement of the ascending aorta. Thorax 1968; 23(4):338–339.

102. David TE, Feindel CM. An aortic valve-sparing operation for patients with aortic incompetence and aneurysm of the ascending aorta. J Thorac Cardiovasc Surg 1992; 103(4):617–621.

103. Yacoub MH, Gehle P, Chandrasekaran V, Birks EJ, Child A, Radley-Smith R. Late results of a valve-preserving operation in patients with aneurysms of the ascending aorta and root. J Thorac Cardiovasc Surg 1998; 115(5):1080–1090.

104. Coady MA, Rizzo JA, Hammond GL, Mandapati D, Darr U, Kopf GS, et al. What is the appropriate size criterion for resection of thoracic aortic aneurysms? J Thorac Cardiovasc Surg 1997; 113(3):476–491.

Chapter 3
Right Heart Valve Disease

Michael Henein

Many of right-sided valve diseases are congenital and once diagnosed they are dealt with early in life. Pulmonary and tricuspid valve disease that develop later in life are either secondary to left-sided heart disease, caused by the same pathology or as part of the natural history of the congenital heart disease.

Right Ventricular Response to Valve Disease

As is the case with the left ventricle the right ventricle responds to pressure overload by hypertrophy and early dilatation. While chronic conditions like pulmonary stenosis and pulmonary hypertension result in early ventricular dilatation, acute pulmonary embolism and consequent increase in afterload does not cause right ventricular dilatation. With the increase in afterload and right ventricular dilatation, the ventricle adapts to increased pressure overload by abducting the interventricular septum to function as part of the right ventricle rather than the left ventricle. This can easily be demonstrated by studying various phases of the cardiac cycle using M-mode echocardiography. Right ventricular dilatation includes the tricuspid annulus and results in tricuspid regurgitation. Eventually the right ventricular systolic function itself

M.Y. Henein (ed.), *Valvular Heart Disease in Clinical Practice*,   155
DOI 10.1007/978-1-84800-275-3_3,

deteriorates, which becomes irreversible even after correcting the volume or pressure overload. With right ventricular volume overload the ventricle is very active, as shown by its free wall movement at the tricuspid ring level. It is generally accepted that assessing right ventricular ejection fraction is difficult because of its complex anatomy, being formed of three components: an inlet portion and an outlet portion which are at a significant angle from each other and the trabecular portion at the apex. The myocardial fiber architecture of the inlet and outlet parts of the right ventricle is significantly different, thus making estimation of the overall systolic function difficult.

Assessment of Right Ventricular Size and Function

While a 3D approach to the assessment of right ventricular systolic function is the ideal way other cross-sectional echocardiographic and cardiac magnetic resonance (CMR) techniques have developed over the years and have proved sensitive in assessing right ventricular ejection fraction. Right ventricular inlet diameter can be used as a marker of cavity dilatation. Free wall long axis movement studied by M-mode and tissue Doppler imaging from the lateral angle of the tricuspid annulus is an easy measure of systolic function and correlates closely with right ventricular ejection fraction, an amplitude less than 20 mm suggests significantly impaired overall systolic function with an ejection fraction of approximately 45%. Likewise, right ventricular outflow tract diameter has been shown to be a sensitive measure of systolic function. In patients with reversed septal movement it is crucial to exclude any shunt as a cause for the volume overload on the right ventricle. Similar measurements can be obtained by CMR based on volumetric changes in systole and diastole. Finally, 3D echocardiography has now proved an ideal tool for assessing overall right ventricular function as well as the contribution of each of its components. Estimation of pulmonary artery pressure is an essential component for examination of patients with right-sided valve disease as well as those limited by breathlessness. The retrograde flow velocity across the tricuspid valve gives an indication of systolic right ventricular pressure using the modified Bernoulli equation $4V^2$. In all patients, systolic pulmonary artery pressure equals the retrograde peak pressure drop across the tricuspid valve added to the estimated right atrial pressure, according to the collapsibility of the inferior vena cava. These measurements are clinically useful in patients with no pulmonary stenosis.

Diagnosis of Valve Stenosis and Regurgitation

The principles used in clinical practice for diagnosing tricuspid and pulmonary valve stenosis and regurgitation are very similar to the ones used in the left side of the heart. Color Doppler detects the level at which there is increased velocities as a sign of valve narrowing and this can be confirmed by continuous wave Doppler. In patients with valve regurgitation, color Doppler assesses the jet diameter, direction and area which, with respect to the right atrial area in cases of tricuspid regurgitation, gives some indication of the severity of tricuspid regurgitation. Transesophageal echo images, particularly in tricuspid valve disease, provide detailed assessment of valve pathology. Transthoracic images of the pulmonary valve can be somewhat limited technically. However, in the majority Doppler excludes significant valve disease based on forward and backward velocities and pressure drop. Transesophageal echo provides a clear image of the pulmonary valve, so ideal for determining the level of valve stenosis. The degree of pulmonary stenosis and regurgitation severity is assessed by continuous wave Doppler. Timing of the pulmonary regurgitation flow reversal is another confirmation for its severity. Mild pulmonary regurgitation occupies the whole of diastole while in severe regurgitation there is early pressure equalization between the two chambers. A jet diameter of 7 mm or more also supports the diagnosis of severe pulmonary regurgitation. CMR is another ideal non-invasive technique for assessment of right-sided chamber size and valve function, in particular the pulmonary valve. The level of narrowing can easily be determined, the degree of stenosis by velocity mapping and severity of regurgitation by estimating the regurgitant volume.

Tricuspid Valve Disease

Anatomy: Morphologically, right atrioventricular valve has three leaflets (tricuspid): septal, inferior (mural) and anterosuperior which are separated from each other by anteroseptal, superoinferior and inferoseptal commissures, respectively. The inferior leaflet takes its origin exclusively from the diaphragmatic parietal wall of the ventricle and is often called the mural leaflet. Each commissure is usually supported by the corresponding papillary muscle. The most characteristic and distinguishing feature of the tricuspid valve is the direct attachment of the cords from the septal leaflet to the septum. These chordal attachments to the septal surface are never seen in the morphological left ventricle except when the tricuspid valve straddles and inserts on the left ventricular septal aspect. The reason for this complex arrangement of chordae tendinae is that the atrioventricular valves must close during systole and these prevent them from ballooning into the atria (Figure 3.1).

Tricuspid Stenosis
Etiology

Tricuspid valve stenosis is less prevalent than mitral stenosis. A number of diseases may contribute to the physiological presentation of tricuspid stenosis.

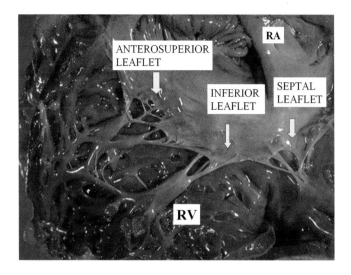

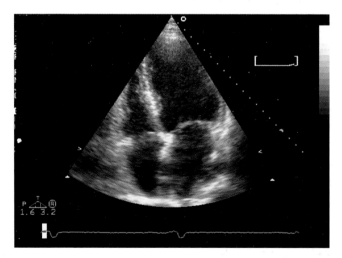

FIGURE 3.1. (top) Section in the right heart showing the anatomy of the tricuspid valve and its relation to the right atrium and ventricle. (bottom) Two-dimensional image of the right heart from the apical view demonstrating the tricuspid septal and anterosuperior leaflets and the trabecular right ventricular apex.

- *Rheumatic valve disease*: This is the most common cause of tricuspid stenosis. The cusps are thickened and the commissures fused so that the valve area becomes small and the valve leaflets dome toward the right ventricle in diastole, similar to rheumatic mitral valve leaflets. In contrast to mitral valve disease, the subvalvar apparatus is not usually involved [1–3] but the annulus may dilate. As the disease progresses, the right atrium dilates and becomes congested. This is always associated with some degree of tricuspid regurgitation Figures 3.2 and 3.3.
- *Carcinoid disease*: This is a colonic tumor that secretes 5-hydroxytryptamine which circulates with the blood and affects usually right heart valves. The tricuspid valve leaflets become fibrosed and fused so that their movement

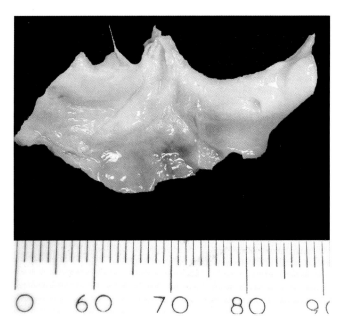

FIGURE 3.2. Pathology section from a patient with rheumatic tricuspid valve leaflets.

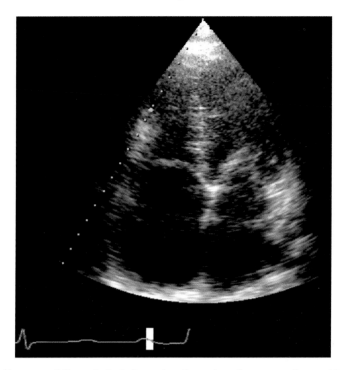

FIGURE 3.3.   Apical four chamber view from a patient with rheumatic mitral and tricuspid valve disease. Note the restricted cusp movement and the valve doming in diastole.

and opening are restricted [4, 5]. Carcinoid disease may affect the mitral valve only in patients with atrial shunts Figures 3.4, 3.5 and 3.6.

– *Right ventricular pacing*: Tricuspid stenosis may infrequently complicate right ventricular pacing. A pacing wire that perforates one of the three leaflets causes local inflammation, fibrosis and leaflet stiffness. This can be missed by echocardiography if right-sided flow velocities are not carefully studied. Color flow Doppler of the tricuspid valve should give an indication of valve narrowing and continuous wave Doppler usually confirms significantly raised

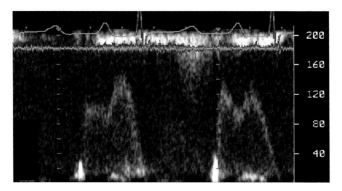

FIGURE 3.4. Continuous wave Doppler across the tricuspid valve from the same patient showing high velocities and a mean pressure drop of 4 mmHg.

forward flow velocities. A severe degree of stenosis caused by pacing wires may require valve replacement and insertion of an epicardial lead [6] Figure 3.6.

– *Functional tricuspid stenosis*: When tricuspid valve leaflets are morphologically normal, raised right ventricular inflow velocities can be caused by a number of pathologies:

a) *A large atrial septal defect*: With significant left to right shunt that increases the right atrial stroke volume, right ventricular filling velocities increase. This does not usually result in conventional signs of tricuspid stenosis. After closure of the atrial septal defect transtricuspid velocities normalize Figure 3.7.

b) *Localized pericardial effusion behind the right atrium*: With progressive increase in a localized effusion pressure the right atrial free wall may collapse and narrow the inflow tract of the right ventricle thus resulting in significantly raised velocities. Irrespective of the volume of the pericardial collection, the localized raised pressure is the direct cause of functional tricuspid stenosis. Draining the pericardial effusion results in complete normalization of valve function and flow velocities Figure 3.8.

c) *Right atrial myxoma*: Although rare with respect to its incidence in the left atrium when present the tumor narrows the right ventricular inflow tract causing raised filling velocities. This disturbed physiology normalizes completely after excision of the tumor.

d) *Right atrial secondaries*: Tumors of different histological entities, ovarian sarcoma, renal carcinoma, lymphoma, etc., may spread hematologically directly to the right atrium. Large right atrial secondaries may occupy a considerable part of the atrium and interfere with right ventricular inflow tract and filling Figures 3.9 and 3.10.

(a)

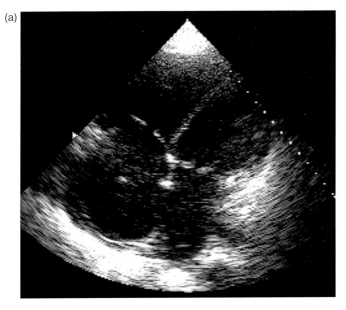

FIGURE 3.5.   (a) Apical four chamber view from a patient with carcinoid tricuspid valve disease showing restricted valve opening in diastole and raised flow velocities. (b) Color flow Doppler of tricuspid valve forward velocities from the same patient demonstrating aliasing (high velocities) at the leaflet level consistent with restricted valve opening and tricuspid regurgitation.

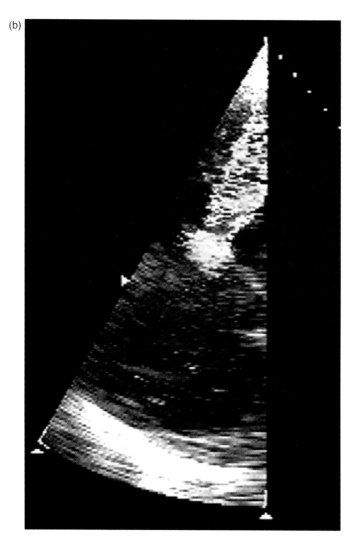

FIGURE 3.5. Continued.

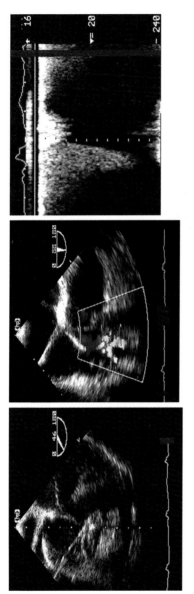

FIGURE 3.6. Transesophageal echo of the right heart showing extensive fibrosis at the site of crossing of the pace-maker leads through the tricuspid valve leaflets. Note the extent of valve fibrosis (*left*) resulting in physiological stenosis shown by aliasing color Doppler (*center*) and raised flow velocities >2 m/s (*right*).

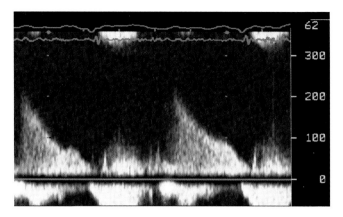

FIGURE 3.7.   Transtricuspid flow velocities from a patient with atrial septal defect. Note the raised velocities up to 2 m/s before closure.

Clinical picture: Regardless of the etiology, the physiological picture of tricuspid stenosis shares a raised transvalvar pressure drop and increased flow velocities. Although this pressure drop is much less than the corresponding one across the mitral valve, it results in raised right atrial pressures and systemic venous congestion of varying severity [7– 9]. Jugular venous pressure is usually raised demonstrating a slow early diastolic descent consistent with high resistance inflow tract of the right ventricle. Long-standing tricuspid stenosis may result in worsening systemic venous congestion, liver dysfunction and ascites. Physical examination may be similar to that of rheumatic mitral stenosis demonstrating an opening snap and a diastolic murmur heard at the right sternal edge which varies with respiration.

Investigations: The chest X-ray shows a large right atrium with normal pulmonary artery size and clear lung fields. Echocardiography is the ideal tool for determining the exact cause of tricuspid stenosis. Conventional 2D imaging helps in assessing right ventricular inflow tract, tricuspid leaflet morphology and function as well as right atrial size. In addition, extra-cardiac causes that may distort the right atrial

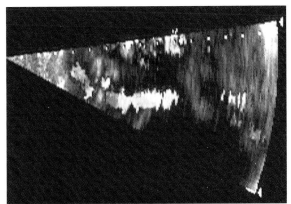

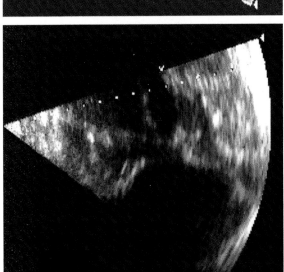

FIGURE 3.8. Apical four chamber view from a patient with localized pericardial effusion behind the right atrium. Note the collapse of the right atrial free wall (*left*) narrowing the inflow tract of the right ventricle and resulting in color aliasing just below the transtricuspid valve level (*right*).

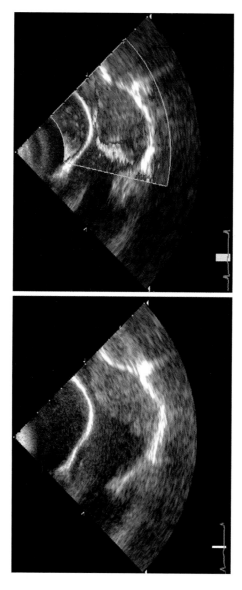

FIGURE 3.9.   Secondaries invading the right atrium resulting in narrowed inflow and high velocities.

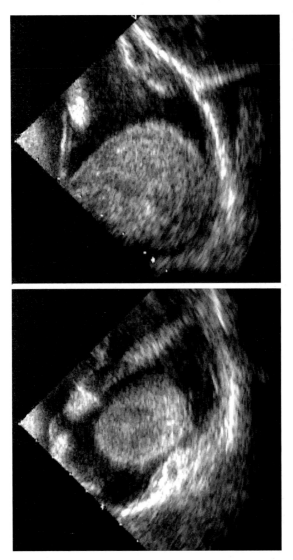

FIGURE 3.10. TOE from a patient with renal cell carcinoma invading the inferior vena cava and the right atrium.

cavity shape and function, e.g., pericardial effusion can be detected. Disturbed normal color flow Doppler pattern along the vertical axis of the right atrium helps in identifying the level of narrowing. This is usually confirmed by pulsed and continuous wave Doppler, particularly when right ventricular filling velocities are raised. Transesophageal echo is ideal for deliniating a clear image of the tricuspid valve leaflets and function. The atrial septum is clearly seen and the extent of tumor invasion of the atrial wall can be assessed. Blood-born tumor spread can also be assessed by careful study of the inferior vena cava on the TOE images of the right atrium.

Treatment: Tricuspid valve disease is a very slowly progressing disease that needs careful follow-up. Mild and moderate tricuspid stenoses are well tolerated. Severe tricuspid stenosis needs surgical repair or replacement if additional regurgitation is present

a) *Medical*: Systemic venous congestion is usually managed with diuretics. However, a balance should be preserved since with the fixed narrowing of the inflow tract right ventricular filling relies on the raised right atrial pressure. Radical cure cannot be achieved without correcting the organic lesion.

b) *Surgical*: Tricuspid valvotomy should be considered at the time of surgery for other valves, particularly with a rheumatic etiology. When missed, it underestimates the surgical success for other lesions, e.g., mitral stenosis. In severe rheumatic tricuspid stenosis, valve replacement is the only option, although this procedure does result in some degree of stenosis from the inserted prosthetic valve. Successful drainage of localized pericardial effusion alleviates the associated functional disturbance. Whenever feasible and appropriate, removal of the right atrial space-occupying lesion (tumor) should result in complete recovery of right heart function as long as it had not invaded the cavity wall.

Tricuspid Regurgitation

Etiology

Mild tricuspid regurgitation is a common finding in 50% normal individuals.

Congenital: The most common cause of congenital tricuspid regurgitation is Ebstein anomaly. The important echocardiographic features of Ebstein malformation are displacement of the hinge point of the septal and mural (inferior) leaflets of the tricuspid valve from the atrioventricular junction into the inlet portion of the right ventricle. In most cases the valve leaflets are dysplastic but in more severe cases the septal or mural leaflets are virtually absent and characteristically the anterosuperior leaflet is large with a so-called 'sail-like' motion. Mild to moderate valve regurgitation is commonly encountered with Ebstein anomaly and an atrial septal defect within the oval fossa usually results in interatrial shunting. Well recognized associated anomalies include not only an atrial septal defect but also pulmonary stenosis and ventricular septal defect. Ebstein malformation of the mitral valve is extremely rare and involvement of the left atrioventricular valve is more likely to be found in congenitally corrected transposition of the great arteries Figures 3.11, 3.12 and 3.13.

– *Functional*: Tricuspid regurgitation frequently occurs with dilatation of the right ventricular cavity and tricuspid ring. It is also seen in patients with pulmonary hypertension irrespective of its etiology or in the terminal stage of congestive heart failure Figure 3.14.

– *Rheumatic disease*: Severe tricuspid regurgitation has been increasingly recognized after mitral valve replacement for rheumatic disease, in the absence of significant left-sided disease or pulmonary hypertension. Recent evidence suggests an organic rheumatic cusp involvement and ring dilatation in this condition [10] Figures 3.15 and 3.16.

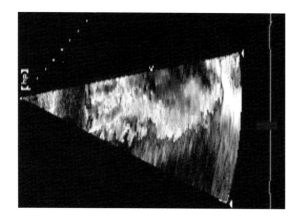

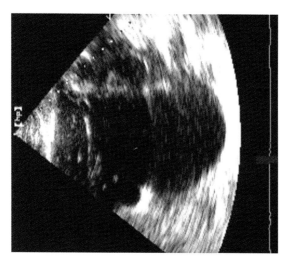

FIGURE 3.11. Apical four chamber view from an adult with Ebstein anomaly and severe tricuspid regurgitation.

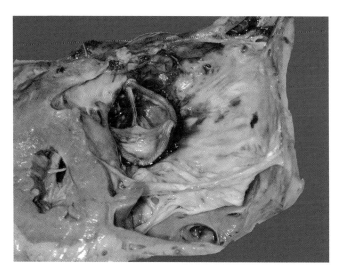

FIGURE 3.12.   Views from the right ventricle showing thickened ballooned and enlarged tricuspid valve leaflets which are displaced down to the right ventricle. There is also a replacement of the mitral valve by a Carpontier Edwards bioprosthesis.

– *Endocarditis*: Isolated tricuspid valve endocarditis is less common than other valves, but when present, it may complicate an infected central line or develop in intravenous drug users [11, 12] Figure 3.17.
– *Endomyocardial fibrosis*: Although rare right-sided endomyocardial fibrosis distorts the inflow tract of the right ventricle and predisposes to severe tricuspid regurgitation. A similar picture is seen with carcinoid syndrome [13] Figures 3.18 and 3.19.
– *Pacemaker insertion*: Significant tricuspid regurgitation may develop as a complication to pacemaker insertion particularly when the lead perforates one of the leaflets. Leaflet fibrosis and retraction develop, resulting in failure of coaption and significant valve incompetence Figure 3.20.

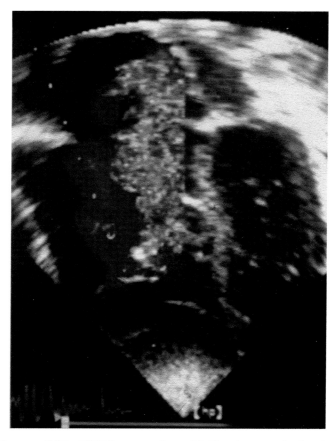

FIGURE 3.13.   TOE from a patient with Ebstein anomaly showing dilated right heart, apical displacement of the septal tricuspid leaflet and severe regurgitation on color flow Doppler.

– *Leaflet prolapse*: Mid-systolic tricuspid valve prolapse may be associated with that of the mitral valve. An example of the association of the two valve dysfunction is seen in Marfan syndrome, although tricuspid regurgitation is usually insignificant compared to mitral regurgitation [14–16] Figure 3.21.

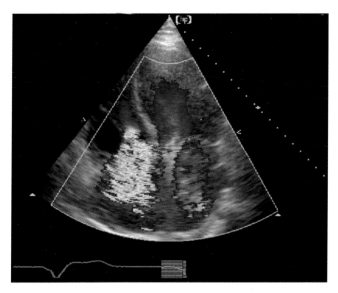

FIGURE 3.14.   Apical four chamber view from a patient with pulmonary hypertension showing dilated right heart and tricuspid regurgitation on color Doppler.

– *Cardiomyopathy*: Long-standing ischemic myocardial disease of the left ventricle may also involve the right ventricle, particularly in patients with prior right ventricular infarction. Progressive ischemic deterioration of the right ventricle may result in dilatation of the basal segment and tricuspid ring and consequently development of significant regurgitation. A similar picture may be seen in late stage of idiopathic dilated cardiomyopathy involving the right heart Figure 3.22.

– *Radiotherapy*: Tricuspid regurgitation is an uncommon complication that may appear many years after radiotherapy to the chest. The exact mechanism of valvular regurgitation is poorly understood Figure 3.23.

Pathophysiology: Mild tricuspid regurgitation is common and does not result in any disturbed hemodynamics. Severe tricus-

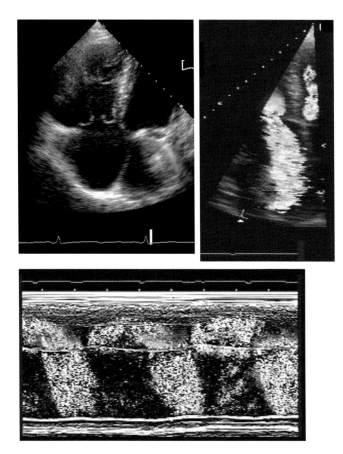

FIGURE 3.15.   Apical views from a patient with rheumatic mitral valve disease showing involved tricuspid leaflets in the disease process. Note the thickened, short and failing to coapt leaflets in systole (*left*) resulting in severe regurgitation on color flow Doppler (*right*) that approaches the back of the right atrium on color flow M-mode (*bottom*).

pid regurgitation, irrespective of its etiology, results in signs and symptoms of raised systemic venous pressure. Raised right atrial pressure is transmitted to the vena cava. A systolic 'V' wave 'from the right ventricle' is seen in the vena cava

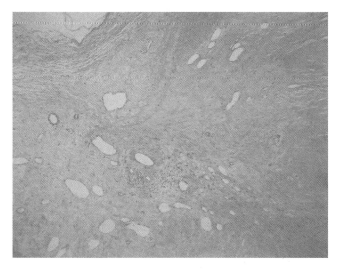

FIGURE 3.16.   Pathological section from a patient with rhematic tricuspid valve disease showing leaflet fibrosis and vascularization.

with the right atrium functioning as a conduit. The systolic wave is followed by a deep wide angled early diastolic 'Y' descent at the time when the tricuspid valve opens and the right ventricle fills (Figure 3.24). Long-standing tricuspid regurgitation results in hepatic congestion and fluid retention and eventually renal impairment. With severe tricuspid regurgitation, the systolic murmur may not be audible due to laminar regurgitation flow.

Clinical Picture

Patients with severe tricuspid regurgitation have raised JVP with prominent V-wave. Expansile pulsation of the liver is present in most cases. The tricuspid regurgitation murmur, when present, is pansystolic and heard at the right sternal edge and is propagated to the epigastrium. It tends to increase in intensity with inspiration as the venous return increases

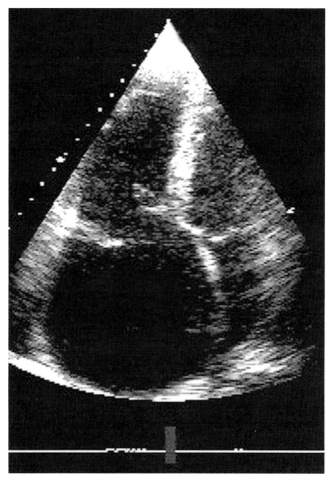

FIGURE 3.17.   Apical 2D views of the right heart from a drug user showing a vegetation attached to the anterosuperior leaflet of the tri-cuspid valve and resulting in leaflet prolapse and failure of coaption.

[17]. Fluid retention is a common finding in most patients with severe regurgitation Figure 3.24.

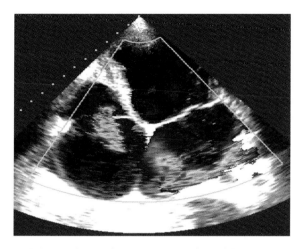

FIGURE 3.18. Apical 2D images from a patient with endomyocardial fibrosis showing distorted right ventricular inlet, fibrosed subvalvar apparatus and tricuspid regurgitation.

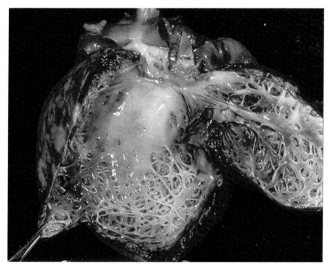

FIGURE 3.19. Pathological section from a patient with endomyocardial fibrosis demonstrating extensive subendocardial fibrosis.

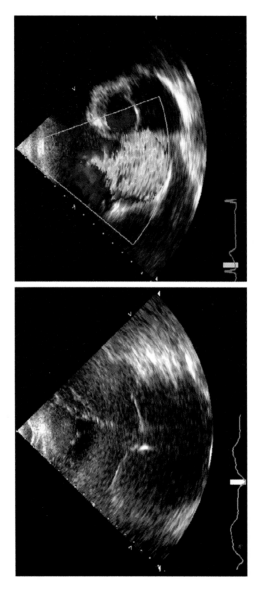

FIGURE 3.20. Apical images from a patient with fluid retention after pacemaker insertion. Note the thickened valve leaflets (*left*) and the severe regurgitation (*right*) resulting from localized fibrosis.

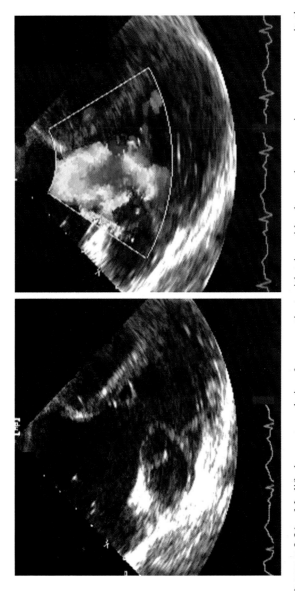

FIGURE 3.21. Modified parasternal view from a patient with tricuspid valve prolapse causing severe regurgitation. Notice the failure of leaflet coaption.

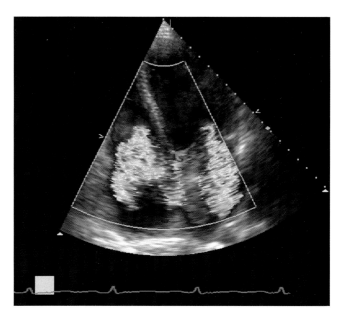

FIGURE 3.22.   Apical four chamber view from a patient with ischemic cardiomyopathy showing dilated four chambers and severe tricuspid regurgitation on the color Doppler picture.

Assessment of Tricuspid Regurgitation

– *Color flow Doppler*: It detects the presence of tricuspid regurgitation, although its absence does not exclude it. A dilated right atrium and a broad regurgitation jet that approaches the vena cava suggest significant incompetence. A tricuspid regurgitation jet area >40% that of the right atrium is consistent with significant regurgitation [18] Figure 3.25.

– *Proximal isovelocity convergence technique*: The same principle as mentioned in the assessment of mitral regurgitation can be applied to determine severity of tricuspid incompetence Figure 3.26.

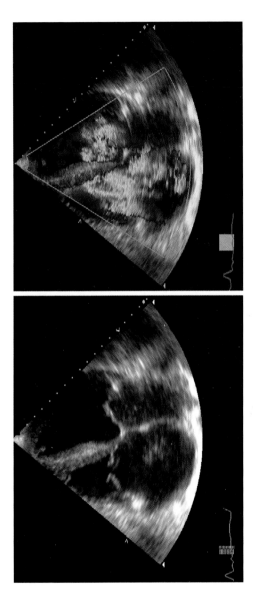

FIGURE 3.23.   Two-dimensional image of the tricuspid valve from a patient, 10 years after radiotherapy. Note the normal looking valve morphology, dilated ring and severe tricuspid regurgitation.

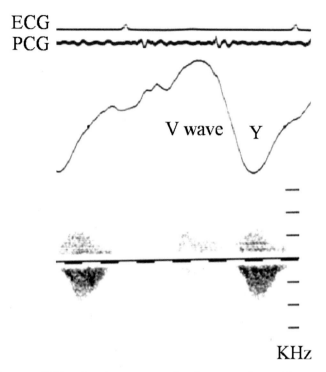

FIGURE 3.24.   Jugular venous pulse from a patient with severe tricuspid regurgitation. Note the prominent systolic 'V' wave on the pulse (*top*) associated with systolic flow reversal in the superior vena cava (*bottom*). This is followed by a deep broad early diastolic 'Y' descent.

- *Continuous wave Doppler*: This registers the pressure drop between the right ventricle and atrium in systole using the modified Bernoulli equation $4V^2$. In the absence of pulmonary valve or infundibular stenosis, adding right atrial pressure (approximately 10 mmHg) to the transtricuspid pressure drop is used to estimate pulmonary artery systolic pressure. Normally with mild functional regurgitation, the higher is the pressure drop across the tricuspid valve the longer it takes to decelerate in early diastole, i.e., after

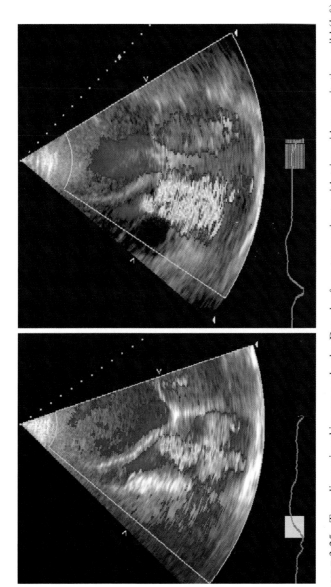

FIGURE 3.25. Two-dimensional images and color Doppler from two patients with tricuspid regurgitation, mild (*left*) and severe (*right*). Note the difference in right atrial size and jet area and diameter.

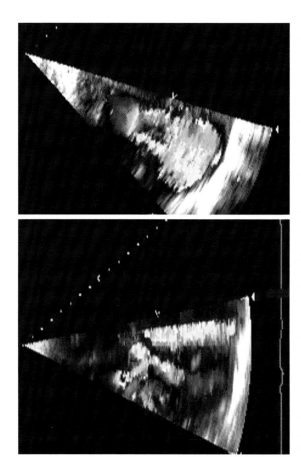

FIGURE 3.26.   Color flow Doppler of severe tricuspid regurgitation from a patient demonstrating PISA technique at the site of leaflet tips.

end-ejection. With severe regurgitation and absence of retrograde tricuspid leaflet resistance, the continuous wave trace becomes more triangular, peaking in early systole and stopping close to end-ejection (P2). This shape represents a reversed V wave in the jugular venous pulse due to pressure equalization between the right atrium and right ventricle at end-ejection. In addition, the pressure drop across the valve may fall to as low as 5–10 mmHg due to the raised right atrial pressure. Equalization of forward and backward flow areas suggests free regurgitation. The combination of this picture along with systolic flow reversal in the superior and inferior venae cavae or hepatic veins and early diastolic forward flow corresponding to the deep Y descent of the venous pulse confirms the diagnosis of severe regurgitation [19–21] Figures 3.27 and 3.28.

– *Reversed septal movement*: With severe right ventricular volume overload from the tricuspid regurgitation the interventricular septal movement becomes reversed and the

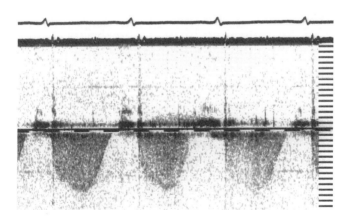

FIGURE 3.27.   Continuous wave Doppler recordings from two patients with tricuspid regurgitation, mild (*left*) and severe (*right*). Note the low pressure drop and the equalization of right ventricular and atrial pressures in early diastole with severe regurgitation.

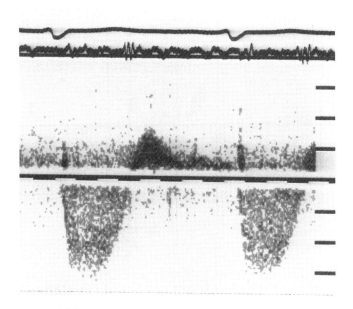

FIGURE 3.27. Continued.

septum functions as part of the right ventricle in systole. This can easily be demonstrated on M-mode images of the left ventricular minor axis Figure 3.29.

Treatment: Many patients tolerate tricuspid regurgitation for a long time, some might present with symptoms that significantly limit their exercise capacity and life-style.

Medical treatment: Diuretics and ACE inhibitors may reduce the systemic venous pressure and improve quality of life for a while. It is always advisable to attempt correcting the tricuspid regurgitation before patients develop irreversible right ventricular damage. Medical treatment may result in significant fall in right ventricular size and hence the extent of tricuspid regurgitation. Moderate to severe regurgitation is reasonably tolerated compared to mitral regurgitation.

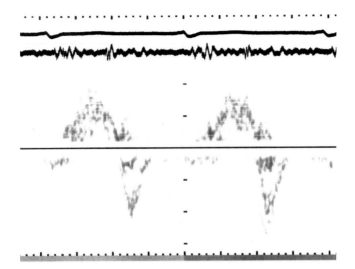

FIGURE 3.28.   Pulsed wave Doppler velocities from a patient with severe tricuspid regurgitation demonstrating flow reversal in the superior vena cava.

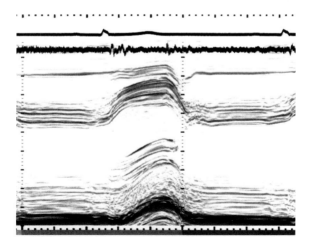

FIGURE 3.29.   M-mode recording of LV minor axis from a patient with severe tricuspid regurgitation demonstrating reversed septal movement.

Tricuspid regurgitation secondary to rheumatic mitral valve disease may subside after successful mitral valve surgery, although direct inspection of the tricuspid valve is always recommended for possible plication and repair in an attempt to avoid future incompetence. If the regurgitation is very severe, and the fluid retention requires very large doses of diuretics large enough to cause significant metabolic consequences, valve repair or replacement may be considered.

Surgical procedures: Tricuspid valve replacement is usually indicated when a prior repair has failed. The repair procedures are less predictable than mitral repair but like the mitral valve it can be performed with or without a supporting ring. Annuloplasty involves either a full ring or an incomplete ring or suture plication of the annulus [22]. The semi-circle ring has the advantage of maintaining the annular flexibility and avoiding conduction disturbances. Residual tricuspid regurgitation occurs less often with the full compared to a semi-circular angioplasty ring [23]. Many young patients with Ebstein anomaly are symptom-free but excellent results of surgical repair have been reported in symptomatic patients. A frequent complication of tricuspid valve replacement is heart block due to the close proximity of the AV node to the tricuspid annulus. It is therefore wise to place permanent epicardial electrodes at the time of surgery. These can be easily connected to a pacing box, thus avoiding the problems of running an endocardial lead through a prosthetic valve. Large right atria are usually complicated by arrhythmia (commonly atrial flutter). Trials to control such arrhythmia by right atrial reduction surgery (Maze operation) have been attempted with good results, particularly in Ebstein anomaly.

Attempts should be made to treat the pulmonary hypertension that is the primary cause of right ventricular dilatation and tricuspid regurgitation. Tricuspid valve replacement by a mechanical prosthesis has a potential risk for endocarditis. Particularly in drug users, bioprostheses have a much lower thrombogenicity and resistance in the tricuspid position and thus may be a preferred choice. The surgical mortality of tricuspid valve surgery is variable between patients and depends particularly on the degree of pre-operative hepatic congestion. Survival following tricuspid valve replacement is not purely related to the surgical procedure itself or to valve function but is significantly affected by right ventricular dysfunction that is almost always masked by the volume overload before surgery.

References

1. Daniels SJ, Mintz GS, Kotler MN. Rheumatic tricuspid valve disease: two-dimensional echocardiographic, hemodynamic, and angiographic correlations. Am J Cardiol 1983; 51(3): 492–496.
2. Guyer DE, Gillam LD, Foale RA, Clark MC, Dinsmore R, Palacios I, et al. Comparison of the echocardiographic and hemodynamic diagnosis of rheumatic tricuspid stenosis. J Am Coll Cardiol 1984; 3(5):1135–1144.
3. Shimada R, Takeshita A, Nakamura M, Tokunaga K, Hirata T. Diagnosis of tricuspid stenosis by M-mode and two-dimensional echocardiography. Am J Cardiol 1984; 53(1):164–168.
4. Pellikka PA, Tajik AJ, Khandheria BK, Seward JB, Callahan JA, Pitot HC, et al. Carcinoid heart disease: clinical and echocardiographic spectrum in 74 patients. Circulation 1993; 87(4):1188–1196.
5. Ross EM, Roberts WC. The carcinoid syndrome: comparison of 21 necropsy subjects with carcinoid heart disease to 15 necropsy subjects without carcinoid heart disease. Am J Med 1985; 79(3):339–354.
6. Heaven DJ, Henein MY, Sutton R. Pacemaker lead related tricuspid stenosis: a report of two cases. Heart 2000; 83(3):351–352.
7. Denning K, Kraus F, Rudolph W. Doppler echocardiography determination of the severity of tricuspid valve stenosis. Herz 1986;11:332–6.
8. Parris TM, Panidis JP, Ross J, Mintz GS. Doppler echocardiographic findings in rheumatic tricuspid stenosis. Am J Cardiol 1987; 60(16):1414–1416.
9. Veyrat C, Kalmanson D, Farjon M, Manin JP, Abitbol G. Noninvasive diagnosis and assessment of tricuspid regurgitation and

stenosis using one and two dimensional echo-pulsed Doppler. Br Heart J 1982; 47(6):596–605.

10. Henein MY, Sheppard M, Ho Y, Pepper J, Gibson DG. Evidence for rheumatic valve disease in patients with severe tricuspid regurgitation long after mitral valve surgery – role of 3D reconstruction. J Heart Valve Dis. In press.

11. Ginzton LE, Siegel RJ, Criley JM. Natural history of tricuspid valve endocarditis: a two dimensional echocardiographic study. Am J Cardiol 1982; 49(8):1853–1859.

12. Bates ER, Sorkin RP. Echocardiographic diagnosis of flail anterior leaflet in tricuspid endocarditis. Am Heart J 1983; 106(1 Pt 1):161–163.

13. Howard RJ, Drobac M, Rider WD, Keane TJ, Finlayson J, Silver MD, et al. Carcinoid heart disease: diagnosis by two-dimensional echocardiography. Circulation 1982; 66(5): 1059–1065.

14. Chandraratna PN, Lopez JM, Fernandez JJ, Cohen LS. Echocardiographic detection of tricuspid valve prolapse. Circulation 1975; 51(5):823–826.

15. Rippe JM, Angoff G, Sloss LJ, Wynne J, Alpert JS. Multiple floppy valves: an echocardiographic syndrome. Am J Med 1979; 66(5):817–824.

16. Schlamowitz RA, Gross S, Keating E, Pitt W, Mazur J. Tricuspid valve prolapse: a common occurrence in the click-murmur syndrome. J Clin Ultrasound 1982; 10(9):435–439.

17. Hansing CE, Rowe GG. Tricuspid insufficiency: a study of hemodynamics and pathogenesis. Circulation 1972; 45(4): 793–799.

18. Suzuki Y, Kambara H, Kadota K, Tamaki S, Yamazato A, Nohara R, et al. Detection and evaluation of tricuspid regurgitation using a real-time, two-dimensional, color-coded, Doppler flow imaging system: comparison with contrast two-dimensional echocardiography and right ventriculography. Am J Cardiol 1986; 57(10):811–815.

19. Currie PJ, Seward JB, Chan KL, Fyfe DA, Hagler DJ, Mair DD, et al. Continuous wave Doppler determination of right ventricular pressure: a simultaneous Doppler-catheterization study in 127 patients. J Am Coll Cardiol 1985; 6(4): 750–756.

20. Sakai K, Nakamura K, Satomi G, Kondo M, Hirosawa K. Hepatic vein blood flow pattern measured by Doppler echocar-

diography as an evaluation of tricuspid valve insufficiency. J Cardiogr 1983; 13(1):33–43.

21. Chan KL, Currie PJ, Seward JB, Hagler DJ, Mair DD, Tajik AJ. Comparison of three Doppler ultrasound methods in the prediction of pulmonary artery pressure. J Am Coll Cardiol 1987; 9(3):549–554.

22. Meyer J, Bircks W. Predictable correction of tricuspid insufficiency by semicircular annuloplasty. Ann Thorac Surg 1977; 23(6):574–575.

23. Rivera R, Duran E, Ajuria M. Carpentier's flexible ring versus De Vega's annuloplasty: a prospective randomized study. J Thorac Cardiovasc Surg 1985; 89(2):196–203.

Chapter 4
Pulmonary Valve Disease

Michael Henein and Wei Li

Anatomy

The pulmonary valve lies anterior and to the left of the aortic valve. The three pulmonary leaflets assume the shape of half moons (semi-lunar) and are similar but usually not equal in size. The right and left coronary sinuses of the aorta always face the pulmonary valve. The leaflets are thinner and more delicate than the aortic leaflets. Unlike the aortic valve, the pulmonary valve sits on a complete muscular ring of the infundibulum and is not in direct continuity with the tricuspid valve. It is thickest along the closing edge. The delicate pocket-like leaflets are formed primarily of collagen and they therefore, open and close passively, with little elastic recoil. In the middle of the free edge of each leaflet is a fibrous mound, the nodule of Arrantius. Coaption of the three nodules ensures complete central closure of the valve orifice during ventricular diastole Figure 4.1.

In adults, the pulmonary valve is better viewed from the parasternal short axis echocardiographic window with anterior angulation Figure 4.2. It can occasionally be seen from the suprasternal and subcostal views. Similar information could be obtained from CMR images of the right ventricular outflow tract. Normal transpulmonary valve blood velocity is in the order of 75 cm/s in mid ejection, which is significantly less than the aortic velocity unless there is left to right shunt [1].

M.Y. Henein (ed.), *Valvular Heart Disease in Clinical Practice*, 195
DOI 10.1007/978-1-84800-275-3_4,
© Springer-Verlag London Limited 2009

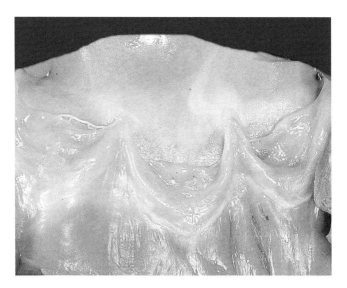

FIGURE 4.1. Section in the right ventricular outflow tract and pulmonary valve showing the three leaflets.

Pulmonary Stenosis

Pulmonary stenosis is a congenital pathology in 95% of cases. It is rarely caused by rheumatic valve disease or carcinoid syndrome. Although it is isolated pathology in most cases it could also be a component of other syndromes, e.g., tetralogy of Fallot. Pulmonary stenosis may take three forms according to the level of outflow tract narrowing: valvar, subvalvar and supravalvar.

(1) Valvular Stenosis

Pulmonary valve stenosis is almost always congenital in origin. It is very rarely rheumatic. Congenital pulmonary stenosis is associated with doming leaflets with total fusion and

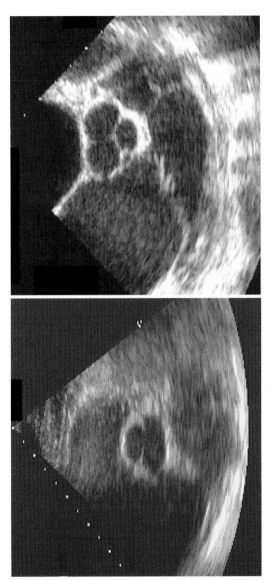

FIGURE 4.2. Short axis view of the aortic valve demonstrating normal looking pulmonary valve leaflets and pulmonary artery diameter. Transthoracic (*left*) and transesophageal (*right*).

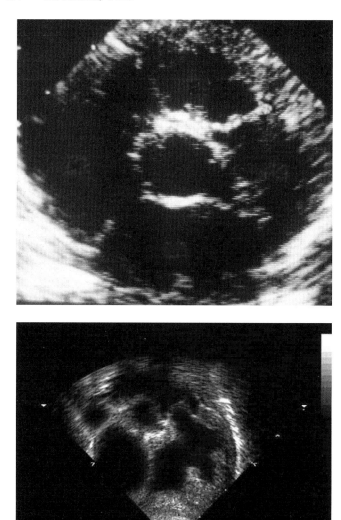

FIGURE 4.3. Subcostal views from a patient with deformed pulmonary valve showing stiff and fibrosed leaflets (*top*) and systolic doming (*bottom*) causing valve stenosis. Pathological section from a patient with bicuspid pulmonary valve.

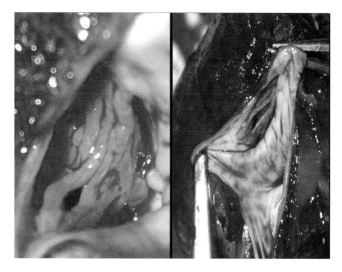

FIGURE 4.3. Continued.

a single orifice in the middle Figure 4.3. In the tetralogy of Fallot, pulmonary valve leaflets are often dysplastic, which are small and thickened and the valve may have only two leaflets [2]. In systole, the leaflets appear doming in the center of the pulmonary artery and are unable to move parallel to the arterial wall as they normally do [3]. In diastole, leaflets may look completely normal since they are not really thickened. Pulmonary stenosis is commonly associated with post stenotic dilatation of the pulmonary artery which itself may suggest the presence of pulmonary stenosis. Contrary to what occurs with the aortic valve, it is uncommon for the pulmonary valve leaflets to calcify with time [4]. Rheumatic pulmonary stenosis is extremely rare. Other rare causes of pulmonary valve stenosis are carcinoid disease [5] where kinins released by the carcinoid tumor in the gastro-intestinal tract cause superficial fibrosis of both the tricuspid and the pulmonary valve.

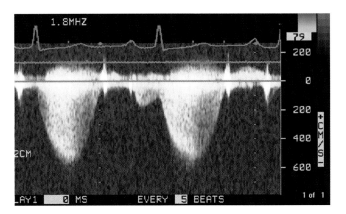

FIGURE 4.4. Continuous wave Doppler velocities across a stenotic pulmonary valve registering a value of 4.5 m/s equivalent to a pressure drop of 81 mmHg.

Pulmonary Stenosis Severity

Color flow Doppler shows the level at which maximum aliasing occurs: valvar, subvalvar or supravalvar. Continuous wave Doppler is the ideal technique for registering peak pulmonary valve velocities that can be translated into a pressure drop by applying the modified Bernoulli equation $4V^2$. A pressure drop of more than 75 mmHg is consistent with severe stenosis [6,7] Figure 4.4. Severe pulmonary stenosis is usually associated with some degree of right ventricular hypertrophy and dysfunction. Significant impairment of right ventricular systolic function and consequently reduction in strok volume may underestimate the severity of pulmonary stenosis when relying solely on the pulmonary velocities and pressure gradient.

(2) Subvalvar Pulmonary Stenosis

Subvalvar pulmonary stenosis is commonly caused by infundibular stenosis or a two chambered right ventricle either in isolation or together with valvar stenosis or Fallot

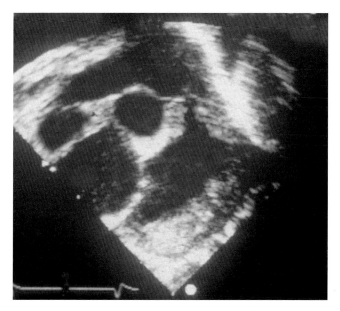

FIGURE 4.5. Subcostal views demonstrating subvalvar (infundibular) pulmonary stenosis. Note the level of narrowing below the valve leaflets.

tetralogy [8]. Subvalvar pulmonary stenosis can easily be seen on 2D images and confirmed by color Doppler Figure 4.5. When it occurs alone, it is often associated with post stenotic dilatation. It may also be part of other disease conditions such as hypertrophic cardiomyopathy that involves the right heart. Rare causes of subvalvar stenosis include tumors, both primary (angiosarcoma or fibroma) and secondary (melanoma) Figure 4.6.

(3) Supravalvar Pulmonary Stenosis

Supravalvar pulmonary stenosis occurs in the proximal segment of the pulmonary artery, either in the form of single or multiple narrowings [9, 10] as in William's syndrome

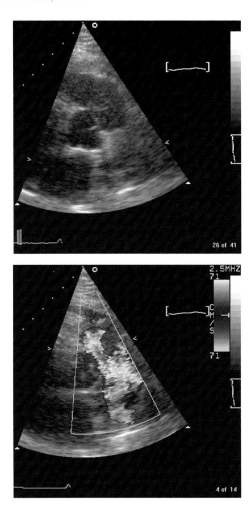

FIGURE 4.6. Parasternal short axis view demonstrating subvalvar pulmonary stenosis caused by secondaries (melanoma).

Figure 4.7. A typical example occurs following banding of the pulmonary artery as part of the management of signifi-cant intracardiac shunting such as multiple ventricular septal

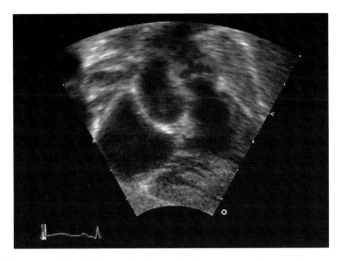

FIGURE 4.7. Subcostal views showing supravalvar pulmonary stenosis of the main pulmonary trunk.

defects [11]. However, supravalvar stenosis may also involve only the pulmonary artery branches and spare the main trunk [12] Figures 4.8 and 4.9. Color flow Doppler indicates the site of narrowing and continuous wave Doppler can be used to assess the severity of stenosis.

Clinical Picture and Management

Patients with mild pulmonary stenosis do not get symptoms. Those with moderate stenosis can tolerate it (pressure drop less than 50 mmHg) for years. Fatigue and dyspnea due to reduced cardiac output are the main symptoms in patients with severe pulmonary stenosis. Physical examination reveals a propagated 'A' wave in the neck and ejection systolic murmur at the upper left sternal edge that radiates to the suprasternal notch and left side of the neck. With severe pulmonary stenosis, the pulmonary component of the second sound may be delayed but often inaudible. An ejection click

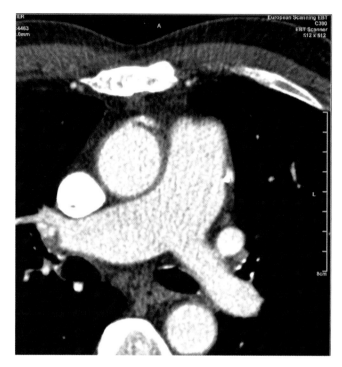

FIGURE 4.8.   Electron beam angiography corresponding to parasternal short axis view from a patient with narrowed left pulmonary artery with respect to a normal right branch.

may be heard at the upper left sternal edge. Event-free survival is closely related to the pressure drop across the pulmonary valve, accounting for 30% for those with a pressure drop above 50 mmHg and 75% for those with a pressure drop less than 50 mmHg.

Balloon valvuloplasty is the ideal procedure for managing congenital pulmonary stenosis in children and early adulthood but the procedure may be complicated by some degree of pulmonary regurgitation [13]. On an average transpulmonary pressure drop falls by two-third the baseline value. Significant regurgitation may develop long after

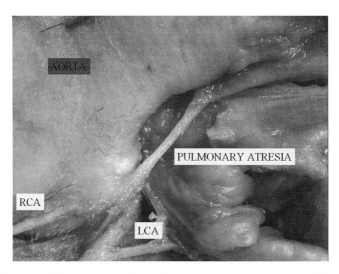

FIGURE 4.9. Section in the pulmonary trunk showing thread-like pulmonary artery, no valve was present at the distal end.

the procedure. Additional subvalvar stenosis may underestimate the success of the procedure. The morbidity rate of this procedure is less than 0.1%. Surgical valvotomy may be considered for patients with failed balloon valvuloplasty. Valve replacement may be needed for patients with iatrogenic significant pulmonary regurgitation, especially after Fallot repair. Homograft replacement might be advantageous to avoid anti-coagulation and thrombogenicity.

Pulmonary Regurgitation

A small amount of pulmonary regurgitation is common in most cases. Significant pulmonary regurgitation is very rare and it is most commonly preceded by intervention to the pulmonary valve during childhood. Although tetralogy of Fallot repair outcome is excellent in most cases, a considerable amount of the developing complications are related to pulmonary regurgitation [14]. Rare causes of pulmonary regurgitation are rheumatic, carcinoid disease and endocarditis. Patients with pulmonary hypertension and dilatation of the right ventricular outflow tract may demonstrate some degree of pulmonary regurgitation. The typical murmur of pulmonary regurgitation is soft diastolic and best heard in the left upper parasternal region. The murmur begins after the pulmonary component of the second sound and may be accompanied by a systolic murmur caused by the increased stroke volume.

Assessment of Pulmonary Regurgitation

1) *Color Doppler*: A jet diameter of more than 7.5 mm is consistent with significant pulmonary regurgitation when compared with CMR assessment [15] Figure 4.10.
2) *Continuous wave Doppler*: Continuous wave Doppler velocities are more accurate in discriminating between mild and significant regurgitation [15]. A pulmonary regurgitation signal that shows a fast deceleration, i.e., pressure equalization, in mid diastole or before the 'Q' wave of the succeeding cycle is consistent with severe regurgitation. Mild regurgitation demonstrates a measurable retrograde pressure drop between the pulmonary artery and the right ventricle in late diastole. Severe pulmonary regurgitation is usually associated with right ventricular dilatation and increased activity in order to accommodate the large stroke volume Figure 4.11.

The degree of pulmonary regurgitation can be assessed using the pulmonary regurgitation index. The pulmonary regurgitation index represents the ratio between the pulmonary regurgitation duration from continuous wave Doppler and total diastolic time expressed as a percent. A pulmonary regurgitation index less than 75% is suggestive of significant regurgitation. In patients with fast heart rate,

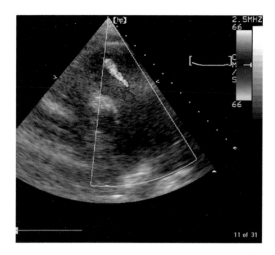

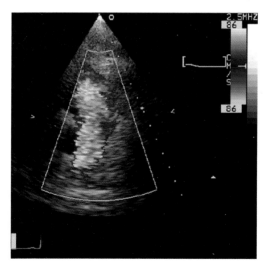

FIGURE 4.10. Parasternal short axis view from two patients with pulmonary regurgitation: mild (*top*) and severe (*bottom*), post pulmonary valvotomy as shown by color flow Doppler. Note the narrow jet in diastole with mild and broad jet (>8 mm) with severe pulmonary regurgitation.

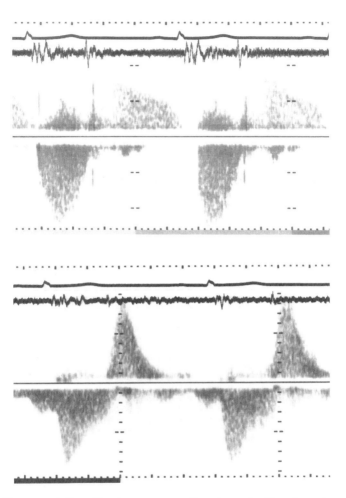

FIGURE 4.11.   Continuous wave Doppler velocities from two patients with pulmonary regurgitation, mild (*top*) and severe (*bottom*). Note the equalization of pulmonary artery and right ventricular pressures in mid diastole in the patient with severe regurgitation.

this index may underestimate the pulmonary regurgitation severity and in those with severe right ventricular disease and raised end-diastolic pressure it may overestimate pulmonary regurgitation severity as the pulmonary artery and right ventricular diastolic pressures will equalize in mid diastole. In patients with atrial fibrillation, an average of five cycles should be considered for estimating pulmonary regurgitation index.

Complications of Pulmonary Regurgitation

1. *Right ventricular dilatation*: Long-standing pulmonary regurgitation is usually well tolerated by the right ventricle, probably due to the low pressure difference between the pulmonary artery and the right ventricular cavity. Even in patients with severe pulmonary regurgitation, the right ventricular cavity may remain completely normal in size and function. However, follow-up of such patients may reveal varying degrees of right ventricular dilatation (remodeling) and eventually dysfunction. Serial measurements of the right ventricular outflow tract diameter (from the long and short axes) and inflow tract (from the apical four chamber view) can be used for monitoring changes in ventricular size in patients with pulmonary regurgitation **Figures** 4.12 and 4.13.

2. *Right ventricular dysfunction*: In some patients with long-standing regurgitation, particularly in the presence of right ventricular dilatation the intrinsic characteristics of the myocardium may change and become stiff (incompliant). The same physiology is frequently observed in patients with small right ventricular size, particularly those with critical pulmonary stenosis and previous valvotomy. In this situation, the right ventricle may not proportionally dilate [16].

3. The features of right ventricular restrictive physiology are (i) an 'A' wave in the pulmonary flow velocity (recorded by pulsed wave Doppler) consistent with direct

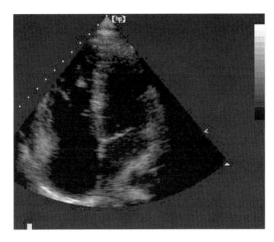

FIGURE 4.12. Apical four chamber view from a patient with severe pulmonary regurgitation showing a slightly dilated right ventricular cavity but maintained function.

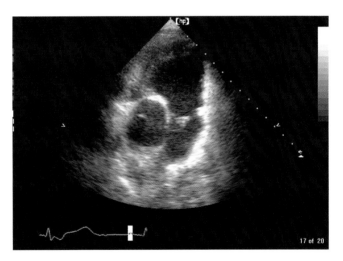

FIGURE 4.13. Short axis of the aortic valve and right ventricular outflow tract demonstrating dilated right ventricle.

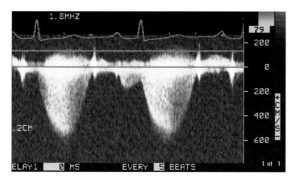

FIGURE 4.14. Transpulmonary continuous wave Doppler from a patient with Noonan's syndrome and pulmonary stenosis showing 'A' wave consistent with restrictive right ventricular physiology. The appearance of an 'A' wave in the pulmonary flow.

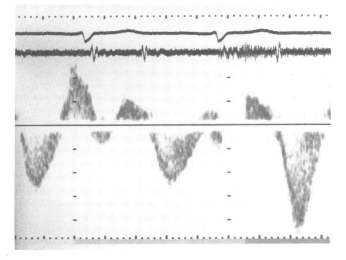

FIGURE 4.15. Superior vena caval flow in the same patient showing giant pressure 'A' wave.

propagation of atrial contraction wave to the pulmonary artery with the right ventricle itself functioning as a conduit in late diastole Figure 4.14; (ii) a giant 'A' wave on Jugular venous pulse Figure 4.15; and (iii) a dominant 'E' wave on

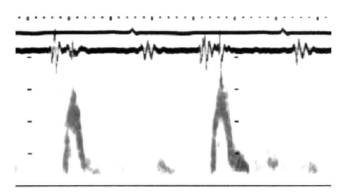

FIGURE 4.16. Right ventricular filling pattern from a patient with restrictive physiology showing dominant 'E' wave with very short deceleration time. Notice the Hwind sound on the planocardiogram at the time of peak E wave.

right ventricular filling pattern with short deceleration time, consistent with raised right atrial pressure Figure 4.16.

Restrictive right ventricular physiology is commonly associated with varying degrees of tricuspid regurgitation and dilatation of the pulmonary artery. Atriogenic tricuspid regurgitation may develop late in the disease process, particularly in patients with a long PR interval that provokes long tricuspid regurgitation. The effect of this advanced ventricular dysfunction is compromised right ventricular filling time and limited stroke volume and exercise intolerance [17]. While similar disturbances on the left side can be corrected by DDD pacing and shortening of the atrioventricular delay, no attempts have been proposed to correct long tricuspid regurgitation that limits right ventricular stroke volume.

3. *Arrythmia*: Untreated significant pulmonary regurgitation may result in atrial or even ventricular arrhythmias. Early correction of the organic valve disease may protect the patient from further deterioration of atrial and ventricular function and subsequent development of arrhythmias Figures 4.17 and 4.18.

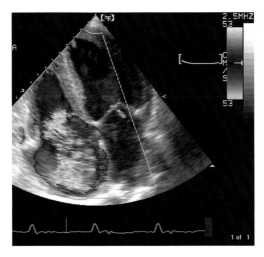

FIGURE 4.17. Apical four chamber view from a patient with right ventricular disease complicated by tricuspid regurgitation as shown by color Doppler.

Assessment of Right Ventricular Function

Quantification of right ventricular function is not always easy because of its complex anatomy. Long axis movement can easily be studied by recording tricuspid ring movement in systole and diastole using M-mode, tissue Doppler or strain and strain rate techniques. Right ventricular free wall (long axis) amplitude has been shown to correlate with overall systolic function assessed by ejection fraction [18]. Also, in early diastole various degrees of functional impairment can be demonstrated by the lengthening velocity and the presence of incoordination (post ejection shortening). Finally, late diastolic amplitude of backward movement of the long axis (toward the atrium) can be used as a marker for assessing right atrial function. Normal right ventricular long axis amplitude is approximately 2.5 ± 0.25 cm [19] Figure 4.19. Myocardial tissue Doppler velocities can be used to assess

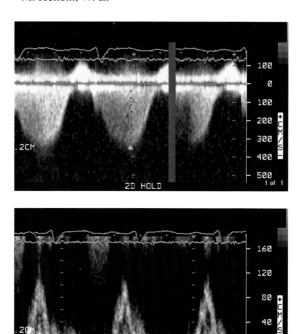

FIGURE 4.18. Continuous wave Doppler from a patient with late stage right ventricular disease demonstrating tricuspid regurgitation with atriogenic component (*top*) that limits total right ventricular filling time (*bottom*).

right ventricular free wall function, again in systole and diastole. Normal values range from 9±2 cm/s for systolic velocity to 10±2 cm/s for early diastolic lengthening velocity.

Complications of Restrictive Right Ventricular Disease

(i) *Cyanosis*: Restrictive right ventricular physiology with increased diastolic pressure results in raised right atrial pressure and possible shunt reversal at atrial level across

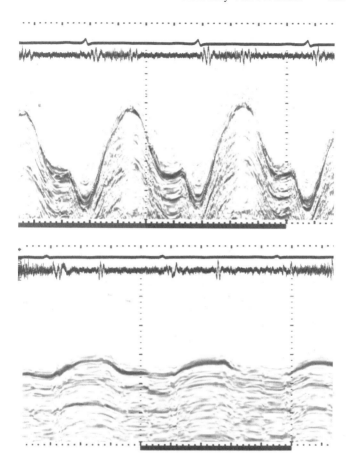

FIGURE 4.19. Right ventricular M-mode recording of free wall long axis from a normal subject (*top*) and a patient with severe right ventricular disease (*bottom*). Note the significant drop in amplitude and velocities, particularly in early diastole.

an atrial septal defect or even a small patent foramen ovale. Patients may experience transient ischemic attacks or cyanosis. Contrast echocardiography with a biological contrast (mixed blood and saline) is often

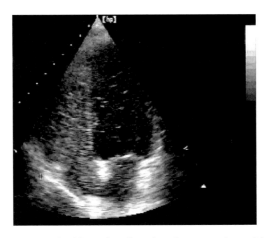

FIGURE 4.20. Apical four chamber view from a patient with restrictive right ventricular disease and cyanosis demonstrating right to left shunt at the atrial level using echo contrast.

useful in confirming the presence of an atrial shunt, particularly with Valsalva maneuvre, when the air bubbles cross the septum and appear in the left atrium Figure 4.20.

(ii) *Right heart failure*: Reduced right ventricular function and increased right atrial pressure will be reflected on the systemic circulation and result in salt and water retention and signs and symptoms of right ventricular decompensation.

(iii) *Arrhythmia:* The increased atrial size and pressure in patients with stiff right ventricle may trigger different forms of arrhythmia: fibrillation or flutter Figure 4.21.

Management

Most patients with mild pulmonary regurgitation remain completely asymptomatic for years. Those with severe

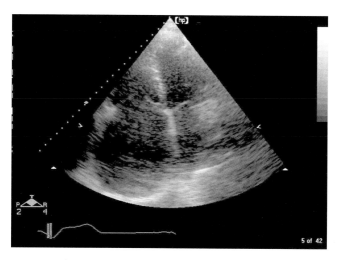

FIGURE 4.21. Apical four chamber view from a patient with stiff right ventricle and arrhythmia demonstrating disproportionately large right atrium.

regurgitation may remain asymptomatic for long time, however, correction of valve incompetence may save them irreversible damage of the right ventricle. Early signs of arrhythmia or progressive right ventricular dilatation are clear indications for surgery. Although pulmonary valve replacement may be a long-term solution for severe pulmonary regurgitation, there is no consensus regarding the exact time for surgical intervention. Decision making should be based on individual cases and considering other factors, e.g., the presence of early signs of right ventricular disease. Pulmonary valve replacement by a homograft has proved a very satisfactory operation with excellent clinical outcome. Transvalvar velocities may be somewhat increased over the early postoperative period but typically remain stable afterward Figure 4.22. With surgical intervention homograft or conduit and valve are used in the pulmonary position. Normalization of right ventricular size and function following pulmonary homograft insertion is not consistent in all patients probably depending on

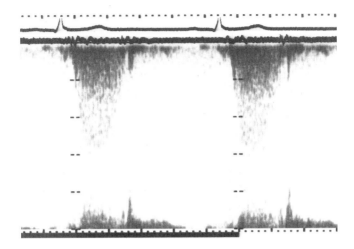

FIGURE 4.22. Continuous wave Doppler recording from a patient with pulmonary homograft 12 months after surgery showing a peak velocity of 2.8 m/s.

pre-operative ventricular dysfunction that could be masked by the volume over-load. Ideally, annual follow-up of these patients should be recommended soon after the first repair.

Recently, transcatheter pulmonary valve replacement has been used and preliminary results are promising [20].

As is the case in restrictive left ventricular physiology, treatment with an ACE – inhibitor may have a substantial role in balancing overall cardiac physiology in patients with restrictive right ventricular disease, but the current literature is lacking the evidence to support this proposal.

References

1. Griffith JM, Henry WL. An ultrasound system for combined cardiac imaging and Doppler blood flow measurement in man. Circulation 1978; 57(5):925–930.
2. Weyman AE, Hurwitz RA, Girod DA, Dillon JC, Feigenbaum H, Green D. Cross-sectional echocardiographic visualization of the stenotic pulmonary valve. Circulation 1977; 56(5):769–774.

3. Leblanc MH, Paquet M. Echocardiographic assessment of valvular pulmonary stenosis in children. Br Heart J 1981; 46(4):363–368.

4. Nishimura RA, Pieroni DR, Bierman FZ, Colan SD, Kaufman S, Sanders SP, et al. Second natural history study of congenital heart defects. Pulmonary stenosis: echocardiography. Circulation 1993; 87(2 Suppl):I73–I79.

5. Pellikka PA, Tajik AJ, Khandheria BK, Seward JB, Callahan JA, Pitot HC, et al. Carcinoid heart disease: clinical and echocardiographic spectrum in 74 patients. Circulation 1993; 87(4):1188–1196.

6. Lima CO, Sahn DJ, Valdes-Cruz LM, Goldberg SJ, Barron JV, Allen HD, et al. Noninvasive prediction of transvalvular pressure gradient in patients with pulmonary stenosis by quantitative two-dimensional echocardiographic Doppler studies. Circulation 1983; 67(4):866–871.

7. Johnson GL, Kwan OL, Handshoe S, Noonan JA, DeMaria AN. Accuracy of combined two-dimensional echocardiography and continuous wave Doppler recordings in the estimation of pressure gradient in right ventricular outlet obstruction. J Am Coll Cardiol 1984; 3(4):1013–1018.

8. Caldwell RL, Weyman AE, Hurwitz RA, Girod DA, Feigenbaum H. Right ventricular outflow tract assessment by cross-sectional echocardiography in tetralogy of Fallot. Circulation 1979; 59(2):395–402.

9. French JW. Aortic and pulmonary artery stenosis: improvement without intervention? J Am Coll Cardiol 1990; 15(7):1631–1632.

10. Wren C, Oslizlok P, Bull C. Natural history of supravalvular aortic stenosis and pulmonary artery stenosis. J Am Coll Cardiol 1990; 15(7):1625–1630.

11. Foale RA, King ME, Gordon D, Marshall JE, Weyman AE. Pseudoaneurysm of the pulmonary artery after the banding procedure: two-dimensional echocardiographic description. J Am Coll Cardiol 1984; 3(2 Pt 1):371–374.

12. Rodriguez RJ, Riggs TW. Physiologic peripheral pulmonic stenosis in infancy. Am J Cardiol 1990; 66(20):1478–1481.

13. Masura J, Burch M, Deanfield JE, Sullivan ID. Five-year follow-up after balloon pulmonary valvuloplasty. J Am Coll Cardiol 1993; 21(1):132–136.

14. Murphy JG, Gersh BJ, Mair DD, et al. Long-term outcome in patients undergoing surgical repair of tetralogy of Fallot. N Engl J Med 1993; 329(9):593–599.

15. Li W, Davlouros P, Gibson DG, Gatzoulis M, Henein MY. Doppler-echocardiographic Assessment of pulmonary regurgitation in adults with repaired tetralogy of Fallot – comparison with cardiovascular magnetic resonance imaging. Am. Heart 2004; 147:165–172. Circulation 2001; 104[II], 431.

16. Hayes CJ, Gersony WM, Driscoll DJ, Keane JF, Kidd L, O'Fallon WM, et al. Second natural history study of congenital heart defects. Results of treatment of patients with pulmonary valvar stenosis. Circulation 1993; 87(2 Suppl):I28–I37.

17. Rowe SA, Zahka KG, Manolio TA, Horneffer PJ, Kidd L. Lung function and pulmonary regurgitation limit exercise capacity in postoperative tetralogy of Fallot. J Am Coll Cardiol 1991; 17(2):461–466.

18. Kaul S, Tei C, Hopkins JM, Shah PM. Assessment of right ventricular function using two-dimensional echocardiography. Am Heart J 1984; 107(3):526–531.

19. Florea VG, Florea ND, Sharma R, Coats AJ, Gibson DG, Hodson ME, et al. Right ventricular dysfunction in adult severe cystic fibrosis. Chest 2000; 118(4):1063–1068.

20. Bonhoeffer P, Boudjemline Y, Saliba Z, Hausse AO, Aggoun Y, Bonnet D, et al. Transcatheter implantation of a bovine valve in pulmonary position: a lamb study. Circulation 2000; 102(7): 813–816.

Chapter 5
Stress Echo in Valvular Heart Disease

Eugenio Picano

Over the last two decades, stress echocardiography has become an established method for evaluating patients with coronary artery disease [1, 2]. While Doppler echocardiography is the method of choice for assessing severity of valvular disease, the role of stress echocardiography has recently expanded to include assessment of hemodynamic consequences of valvular lesions during stress [3–5]. In a number of clinical conditions, particularly in patients with low-gradient, low-flow aortic stenosis, the use of stress echocardiography in the decision-making process has significantly modified the clinical outcome. Evidence accumulated over the last 5 years led to the incorporation of stress echocardiography in the guidelines of the American Heart Association/American College of Cardiology [6], European Society of Echocardiography [7], The American Society of Echocardiography [8] and The European Association of Echocardiography [9]. On the basis of the recent recommendations of these scientific organizations, the use of stress echocardiography in valve disease, according to the published evidence, has been ranked as shown in Table 5.1. Applications are either 'proven' (three stars in the table), 'probable' (two stars) or 'possible but not yet established' (one star) value. Indications of 'proven useful' have been incorporated in either one or more of the general cardiology guidelines [6, 7]; of 'probable usefulness' in general guidelines or stress echo special recommendations [8, 9] but of 'possible value' is not supported

M. Henein (ed.), *Valvular Heart Disease in Clinical Practice*,
DOI 10.1007/978-1-84800-275-3_5,
© Springer-Verlag London Limited 2009

TABLE 5.1. Stress echocardiography applications in valvular heart disease

Target	Tools				
	Aortic gradients (CW)	EF (2D)	Mitral gradient (CW) PASP (CW)	MR (color) PASP (CW)	Transprosthesis gradient (CW)
Aortic stenosis					
Low-gradient, low-flow	***				
High-gradient, high-flow	*				
Aortic regurgitation					
Asymptomatic, severe LV dysfunction		*			
Mitral stenosis					
Symptomatic, mild			***		
Asymptomatic, severe			***		
Mitral regurgitation					
Symptomatic, mild				**	
Asymptomatic, severe				***	
Valve prosthesis					
Symptomatic, equivocal rest findings					**

***=AHA/ACC and/or ESC guidelines; **=ASE and/or EAE recommendations; *=promising reports; color= color Doppler; CW=continuous wave Doppler; PASP=pulmonary artery systolic pressure (from tricuspid regurgitant jet velocity); PW=pulsed wave Doppler.

by the guidelines since it is based only on initial, encouraging experience reported in the literature. The applications of 'proven value' should be implemented in daily clinical practice; the applications of 'probable value' can be implemented in selected cases and the applications of 'possible value' remain limited to research interest only and pertaining to the research domain today.

Aortic Stenosis with Low-Gradient and Left Ventricular Dysfunction

Patients with severe aortic stenosis and low-cardiac output (ejection fraction <40%) often present with a relatively low-pressure gradient, i.e., mean gradient <40 mmHg (Figure 5.1). Such patients can be difficult to distinguish from those with low-cardiac output because of pump failure, and only mild to moderate aortic stenosis. In the former (true anatomically severe aortic stenosis), the small valve area contributes to a raised afterload, decreased ejection fraction and low-stroke volume. In the latter, myocardial contractile dysfunction is primarily the cause of the compromised ejection fraction and low-stroke volume; the problem is further complicated by reduced valve opening forces that contribute to limited valve mobility and apparent stenosis. In both situations, the low-flow state and low-pressure gradient contribute to a calculated effective orifice area that meets criteria for severe aortic stenosis, at rest. In selected patients with low-flow/low-gradient aortic stenosis and left ventricular dysfunction, it may be useful to determine the transvalvular pressure gradient and to calculate valve area during a baseline state and again during low-dose pharmacological (i.e., dobutamine infusion) stress, aiming to determine whether stenosis is severe or only moderate in severity [10, 11–17]. Such studies are usually performed in the echocardiography laboratory. This approach is based on the notion that patients who do not have true anatomically

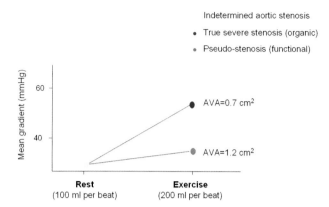

FIGURE 5.1.   Hemodynamics behind the use of dobutamine stress echo in low-gradient aortic stenosis. Below a mean gradient is low regardless of AVA (aortic valve area), conversely, a low calculated AVA does not necessarily indicate anatomically severe aortic stenosis (*yellow dot* at baseline). The stroke volume on the X-axis is low at rest (35 ml) and may normalize following dobutamine (50 ml). The compromised stroke volume may overestimate the degree of valve stenosis, thus making AVA flow dependent. The graph shows the relationship between mean pressure gradient and transvalvular flow for two fixed values of AVA representing mild (>1.5 cm^2, *green dot* following dobutamine) and severe (<1.0 cm^2, *red dot* following dobutamine) stenosis. Modified from Grayburn, 2006 [11].

severe stenosis will exhibit an increase in the valve area and little change in transvalvular gradient in response to an increase in stroke volume [11, 12] Figure 5.2. Thus, if dobutamine infusion produces an increment in stroke volume and an increase in valve area greater than 0.2 cm^2 and little change in gradient, it is likely that baseline evaluation were consistent with non-significant aortic stenosis (Figure 5.3). In contrast, patients with severe aortic stenosis will have a fixed valve area with an increase in stroke volume and an increase in gradient (Figure 5.4) Table 5.2. These patients are likely to improve symptomatically with aortic valve replacement. Patients who fail to show an

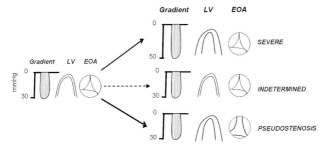

FIGURE 5.2.   Pathophysiology behind dobutamine stress echo in low-gradient aortic stenosis with left ventricular dysfunction. On the left, resting transaortic gradient (<40 mmHg) and left ventricular function (<40%) with calculated effective orifice area (<1 cm^2). On the right, the three possible responses after dobutamine challenge: the increase in stroke volume (>20%) leads to increase in gradients and no increase in effective orifice area in true fixed stenosis, but to only mild increase in gradient and increase in effective orifice area in 'pseudostenosis'. The stenosis remains 'indeterminate' when there is no inotropic response of the left ventricle.

increase in stroke volume with dobutamine (less than 20%), referred to as 'lack of contractile reserve', are known to have a poor prognosis with either medical or surgical management [18]. Dobutamine stress testing in patients with aortic stenosis should be performed only in centers with experience in pharmacological stress testing and with a cardiologist in attendance. Although patients with low-output severe aortic stenosis have a poor prognosis, in those with contractile reserve, outcome is still better with aortic valve replacement than with medical therapy [19]. A number of those without contractile reserve may also benefit from aortic valve replacement, but decisions in these high-risk patients must be individualized, in the absence of clear guidelines. In such patients, the indication for dobutamine stress echo is rated as class IIa, with level of evidence B [6].

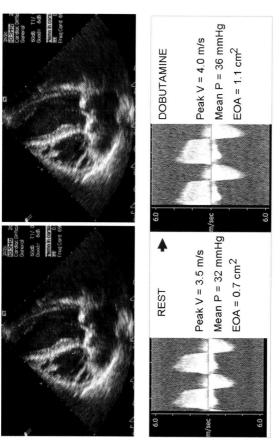

FIGURE 5.3. A typical case of pseudo aortic stenosis unmasked by dobutamine stress echo in a patient with reduced left ventricular function and low-gradient at rest.

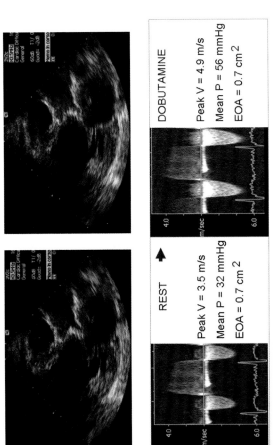

FIGURE 5.4. A typical case of aortic truestenosis unmasked by dobutamine stress echo in a patient with reduced left ventricular function and low-gradient at rest.

TABLE 5.2. Dobutamine stress echo in low-gradient, low-flow aortic stenosis

	Severe AS	Pseudostenosis	Indeterminate
Aortic valve area	No change	Increase ≥ 0.3 cm^2	No change
Mean pressure gradient	Markedly increased	No change	No change
Stroke volume >20%	Yes	Yes	No

Asymptomatic Aortic Stenosis with High-Gradient

As shown in Figure 5.1, the transvalvular aortic gradient increases with increasing flow rates, the higher the transvalvular flow, the higher the pressure gradient. This led to the proposal of exercise stress echo in asymptomatic patients with severe aortic stenosis, defined as peak velocity >4 m/s and/or mean pressure gradient >40 mmHg and/or effective orifice area <1 cm^2 [20]. Management of asymptomatic patients with aortic stenosis remains a source of debate. The wide variation in their individual outcome has recently raised the question of early elective surgery. In this respect, exercise testing is an important tool, and several studies have shown its prognostic value. A reduced exercise tolerance, with development of dyspnoea or ST segment depression, is associated with a worse outcome. On the top of this well established knowledge, a mean pressure gradient rise >20 mmHg may contribute to a worse prognosis and possibly favors early valve replacement [20]. More confirmatory data are needed to support the incorporation of this parameter in the daily management of asymptomatic patients with high-gradient aortic stenosis.

Aortic Regurgitation

As is the case with chronic mitral regurgitation, development of irreversible left ventricular dysfunction is a major concern in asymptomatic patients with severe aortic regurgitation. In those with normal resting left ventricular function, a stress, exercise or pharmacological, induced increase in contractile reserve before surgery may predict improvement in left ventricular function after valve replacement procedure. The use of contractile reserve measurements can be extended for the evaluation of patients with aortic regurgitation who had developed left ventricular dysfunction. The validity of stress echocardiography in this setting is limited mainly by the small number of available studies [21, 22]. To this effect, the ACC/AHA guidelines do not recommend exercise or dobutamine stress echocardiography for routine assessment of left ventricular function in patients with aortic regurgitation. More data are needed to corroborate this application, since the incremental value of stress data to left ventricular dimensions and ejection fraction at rest remains unclear [8]. The observed magnitude of change in ejection fraction from rest to exercise is related not only to myocardial contractile function but also to severity of volume-overload and exercise-induced changes in preload and peripheral resistances [6].

Mitral Stenosis and Discordant Symptoms and Stenosis Severity

A baseline resting transthoracic echocardiography examination is usually enough for dictating management in asymptomatic patients with mild mitral stenosis and in symptomatic patients with moderate-to-severe stenosis, who are candidates for either percutaneous or surgical mitral valve repair. In some patients, more detailed assessment of valve function and its hemodynamic consequences, particularly when symptoms and Doppler findings are not matching, is needed.

In asymptomatic patients with severe stenosis (mean gradient >10 mmHg and mitral valve area <1.0 cm^2) or symptomatic patients with moderate stenosis (mean gradient of 5–10 mmHg and mitral valve area of 1.0–1.5 cm^2), the measurement of pulmonary pressures during exercise may help distinguish those who could benefit from surgery from those who should continue on medical therapy [23–25]. As is the case with the aortic valve (Figure 5.1), transmitral valve pressure gradient is related to the valve orifice area. The usually adopted cut-off values, proposed by the ACC/AHA guidelines [6], are a rise of >60 mmHg for peak systolic pulmonary artery pressure (from the tricuspid regurgitant velocity) during exercise or >15 mmHg mean transmitral pressure gradient (from transmitral flow velocities) Figure 5.5 [6]. Above this threshold, valve repair is recommended, even for symptomatic mitral stenosis with moderate severity at rest [6, 8, 9]. Stress echo application in mitral stenosis with discordant symptoms and stenosis severity is rated as class I with level of evidence C [6].

Mitral Regurgitation

Assessment of mitral regurgitation is qualitatively and semi-quantitatively achieved by color Doppler technique [6, 7]. Such information is usually quite satisfactory in explaining symptoms in patients with significant mitral regurgitation and volume overload and there is seldom a need for further assessment of valve and ventricular function during stress. In selected cases with discrepancy between symptoms and severity of valve regurgitation, e.g., asymptomatic patients with severe mitral regurgitation, stress echocardiography may prove a useful tool to identify patients with a poor prognosis. The spectrum of left ventricular response to stress is not dissimilar from that described for aortic insufficiency—but the prognostic impact of this functional heterogeneity remains unsettled. The rise of pulmonary artery systolic

REST   STRESS

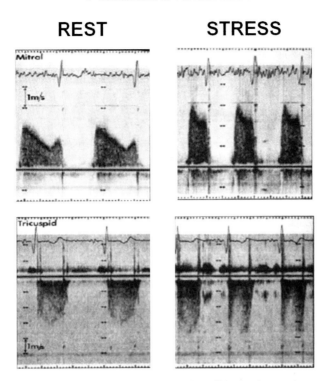

FIGURE 5.5. A symptomatic patient with mild mitral stenosis at rest (mean gradient 5 mmHg) develops a severe stenosis (mean gradient 18 mmHg) with pulmonary systolic arterial pressure >60 mmHg during semi-supine exercise, suggesting a need for mitral valve repair. Modified from Ref. [3].

pressure during exercise/stress >60 mmHg unmasks patients with latent left ventricular dysfunction who might be referred to surgery [6, 8]. Exercise echocardiography has been used to uncover the development of severe mitral regurgitation, with exercise, in patients with rheumatic mitral valve disease and only mild mitral stenosis and regurgitation at rest [26]. Likewise, exercise echocardiography is valuable in identifying hemodynamically significant mitral regurgitation in patients with left ventricular systolic dysfunction, e.g., particularly when ischemia is the underlying etiology. In some patients, dynamic mitral regurgitation can cause acute pulmonary edema and predicts poor outcome [27]. Those patients who develop an increase of effective regurgitant orifice or systolic pulmonary pressure at peak stress are known to have a higher incidence of morbidity and mortality [27]. Stress echo application in asymptomatic severe mitral insufficiency is rated as class IIa with level of evidence C [6].

Valve Prostheses

When prosthetic valve dysfunction is suspected, a careful history and physical examination is vital. Rarely, if transthoracic and, when needed, transesophageal echocardiography or cinefluoroscopy studies are not informative in a patient with exertional symptoms, exercise stress echocardiography may be needed to assess the valve prosthesis function at higher cardiac output [28]. A disproportionate ($>$100%) rise of transvalvular gradient suggests prosthesis dysfunction [29–36]. Despite its use in determining efficient valve function, most studies do not show a convincing correlation between valve size, resting and exercise gradients and exercise tolerance [34–36]. There is also contradictory evidence linking high gradients with a higher risk of death and other complications [37–40]. Further studies are needed in this challenging field.

Diagnosis of Coronary Artery Disease in Patients with Valvular Heart Disease

Although stress echocardiography is a widely accepted, accurate, radiation-free and safe technique to detect the presence of significant coronary artery disease non-invasively in patients without valvular disease, relatively few data are available on its accuracy and safety in patients with significant valvular problems. In general, one can expect that the sensitivity of stress echocardiography will be similar in patients with and without valvular heart disease but the specificity will be lower [41]. In fact, coronary flow reserve can be severely reduced in patients with aortic stenosis or aortic insufficiency even when the coronary arteries are completely smooth [41]. For this same reason, the specificity of perfusion changes is lower than wall motion changes in patients with left ventricular hypertrophy secondary to valvular heart disease [42]. For practical purposes, conventional coronary angiography remains an established investigation to rule out significant coronary disease in the pre-surgical evaluation of these patients.

Coronary Flow Reserve in Patients with Valvular Heart Disease

Coronary flow reserve may be impaired in patients with severe aortic stenosis, in a way largely independent of left ventricular hypertrophy, possibly due to increased left ventricular end-diastolic pressure and concomitant coronary microvascular disease [43–46]. Following aortic valve replacement normalization of coronary flow reserve is more frequently observed with stentless valves, probably posing less hemodynamic burden on the left ventricle both at rest and during exercise [45]. In the future, the assessment of coronary flow reserve on mid-distal left anterior descending coronary artery by transthoracic stress echocardiography is likely to play an increasing role in ventricular functional characterization in the presence of native valve disease, especially the aortic valve [46], and its remodeling following valve replacement (Figure 5.6). Interesting data have been obtained by PET [44] and CMR [45] in this field, but the obvious advantage of transthoracic vasodilator stress echocardiography and its wide availability, low-cost (and lack of substantial radiation exposure when compared to PET) make it a superior alternative [47, 48].

6 months post-AVR

Pre-AVR

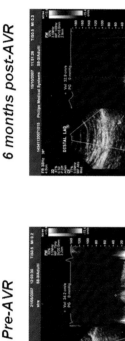
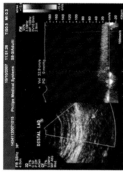
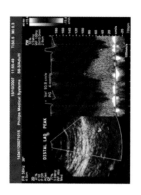
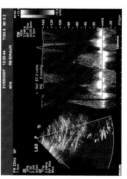
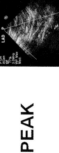

REST

PEAK

FIGURE 5.6. Coronary flow reserve detected by transthoracic stress echocardiography in a patient with severe aortic stenosis and angiographically normal coronary arteries before (*left panel*) and 1 week after (*right panel*) aortic valve replacement. In the post-operative assessment, left ventricular hypertrophy is not yet regressed but coronary flow reserve has substantially improved, possibly as a result of decreased endoventricular diastolic compressive forces. Courtesy of Dr Fausto Rigo, Venice, Italy.

Conclusions

Stress echocardiography has an established role in the clinical decision-making of patients with valvular heart disease. Surprisingly, this role is much more clearly established in American [6] than European [7] general cardiology guidelines—in spite of the larger and earlier acceptance of stress echocardiography in the European practice for the diagnosis of coronary artery disease [1, 9]. There is little doubt that the role of stress echo in valvular heart disease has now become an integral component [7, 8] Table 5.3. The radiation-free, low-cost and tremendously versatile nature of stress echo information ranges from left to right ventricular function, pulmonary hemodynamic, coronary flow reserve, valve gradient and incompetence. Such versatility seems ideally suited for a tailored application in the individual valvular heart disease. In addition, Doppler parameters employed in stress echo for valvular heart disease are, in general, simpler to obtain and more amenable to quantification com-

TABLE 5.3. Stress echo applications in coronary and valvular heart diseases

Diagnostic target	CAD	Valvular
Present application	Dominant	Marginal
Expected rise	+++	+++
Technique	2D	PW, CW, 2D, color
Diagnostic end-point	Regional wall motion	Gradients, pressures, insufficiency, LV function
Approach	One fits all	Tailored on patient
Stress	Exercise, DIP, DOB	Exercise or DOB
Analysis	Qualitative	Quantitative

Abbreviations: CAD=coronary artery disease; CW= continuous wave Doppler; DIP= dipyridamole; DOB= dobutamine; PW=pulsed Doppler; +++=three-fold increase in the next 5 years.

pared with the eyeballing regional wall motion analysis which remains the cornerstone of coronary artery disease diagnosis [1, 7, 8].

References

1. Picano E. Stress echocardiography: from pathophysiological toy to diagnostic tool. Point of view. Circulation 1992; 85:1604–1612.
2. Fox K, Garcia MA, Ardissino D, Buszman P, Camici PG, Crea F, Daly C, De Backer G, Hjemdahl P, Lopez-Sendon J, Marco J, Morais J, Pepper J, Sechtem U, Simoons M, Thygesen K, Priori SG, Blanc JJ, Budaj A, Camm J, Dean V, Deckers J, Dickstein K, Lekakis J, McGregor K, Metra M, Morais J, Osterspey A, Tamargo J, Zamorano JL. Task Force on the Management of Stable Angina Pectoris of the European Society of Cardiology; ESC Committee for Practice Guidelines (CPG). Guidelines on the management of stable angina pectoris: executive summary: the Task Force on the Management of Stable Angina Pectoris of the European Society of Cardiology. Eur Heart J 2006; 27:1341–1348.
3. Schwammenthal E, Vered Z, Rabinowitz B, Kaplinsky E, Feinberg MS. Stress echocardiography beyond coronary artery disease. Eur Heart J 1997; 18:D130–D137.
4. Decena BF III, Tischler MD. Stress echocardiography in valvular heart disease. Cardiol Clin 1999; 17:555–572
5. Fulps D, Davis C, Shah P. Exercise Doppler echocardiography: utility in obtaining hemodynamic evaluation. Cardiac Ultrasound Today 2002; 7/8: 118–149.
6. Bonow RO, Carabello BA, Chatterjee K, de Leon AC, Jr., Faxon DP, Freed MD, Gaasch WH, Lytle BW, Nishimura RA, O'Gara PT, O'Rourke RA, Otto CM, Shah PM, Shanewise JS, Smith SC, Jr., Jacobs AK, Adams CD, Anderson JL, Antman EM, Fuster V, Halperin JL, Hiratzka LF, Hunt SA, Lytle BW, Nishimura R, Page RL, Riegel B. ACC/AHA 2006 guidelines for the management of patients with valvular heart disease: a report of the American College of Cardiology/American Heart Association Task Force on Practice Guidelines (writing Committee to Revise the 1998 guidelines for the management of patients with valvular heart disease) developed

in collaboration with the Society of Cardiovascular Anesthesiologists endorsed by the Society for Cardiovascular Angiography and Interventions and the Society of Thoracic Surgeons. J Am Coll Cardiol 2006; 48:e1–148.

7. Vahanian A, Baumgartner H, Bax J, Butchart E, Dion R, Filippatos G, Flachskampf F, Hall R, Iung B, Kasprzak J, Nataf P, Tornos P, Torracca L, Wenink A. Task Force on the Management of Valvular Heart Disease of the European Society of Cardiology; ESC Committee for Practice Guidelines. Guidelines on the management of valvular heart disease: The Task Force on the Management of Valvular Heart Disease of the European Society of Cardiology. Eur Heart J 2007; 28: 230–268.

8. Pellikka PA, Nagueh SF, Elhendy AA, Kuehl CA, Sawada SG. American Society of Echocardiography: American Society of Echocardiography recommendations for performance, interpretation, and application of stress echocardiography. J Am Soc Echocardiogr 2007; 20:1021–1041.

9. Sicari R, Nihyoannopoulos P, Evangelista A, Kasprzak, Lancelotti P, Poldermans D, Voigt JU, Zamorano JL. European Association of Echocardiography. Stress echocardiography expert consensus statement: European Association of Echocardiography (EAE) (a registrered branch of the ESC). Eur J Echocardiogr. 2008; 9:415–437.

10. Otto CM, Pearlman AS, Kraft CD, Miyake-Hull CY, Burwash IG, Gardner CJ. Physiologic changes with maximal exercise in asymptomatic valvular aortic stenosis assessed by Doppler echocardiography. J Am Coll Cardiol 1992; 20:1160–1167.

11. Grayburn PA. Assessment of low-gradient aortic stenosis with dobutamine. Circulation 2006; 113:604–606.

12. deFilippi CR, Willett DL, Brickner ME, et al. Usefulness of dobutamine echocardiography in distinguishing severe from non severe valvular aortic stenosis in patients with depressed left ventricular function and low transvalvular gradients. Am J Cardiol 1995; 75:191–194.

13. Bermejo J, Garcia-Fernandez MA, Torrecilla EG, et al. Effects of dobutamine on Doppler echocardiographic indexes of aortic stenosis. J Am Coll Cardiol 1996; 28:1206–1213.

14. Lin SS, Roger VL, Pascoe R, Seward JB, Pellikka PA. Dobutamine stress Doppler hemodynamics in patients with aortic stenosis: feasibility, safety, and surgical correlations. Am Heart J 1998, 136:1010–1016.

15. Monin JL, Monchi M, Gest V, Duval-Moulin AM, Dubois-Rande JL, Gueret P. Aortic stenosis with severe left ventricular dysfunction and low transvalvular pressure gradients: risk stratification by low dose dobutamine echocardiography. J Am Coll Cardiol 2001; 37: 2101–2107.

16. Schwammenthal E, Vered Z, Moshkowitz Y, et al. Dobutamine echocardiography in patients with aortic stenosis and left ventricular dysfunction: predicting outcome as a function of management strategy. Chest 2001; 119:1766–1777.

17. Nishimura RA, Grantham JA, Connolly HM, Schaff HV, Higano ST, Holmes DR, Jr. Low-output, low-gradient aortic stenosis in patients with depressed left ventricular systolic function: the clinical utility of the dobutamine challenge in the catheterization laboratory. Circulation 2002; 106:809–813.

18. Monin JL, Quere JP, Monchi M, et al. Low-gradient aortic stenosis: operative risk stratification and predictors for long-term outcome: a multicenter study using dobutamine stress hemodynamics. Circulation 2003; 108:319–324.

19. Burwash IG. Low-flow, low-gradient aortic stenosis: from evaluation to treatment. Curr Opin Cardiol 2007; 22:84–91.

20. Lancellotti P, Lebois F, Simon M, Tombeux C, Chauvel C, Pierard LA. Prognostic importance of quantitative exercise Doppler echocardiography in asymptomatic valvular aortic stenosis. Circulation 2005; 112:I377–I382.

21. Wahi S, Haluska B, Pasquet A, Case C, Rimmermann CM, Marwick TH. Exercise echocardiography predicts development of left ventricular dysfunction in medically and surgically treated patients with asymptomatic severe aortic regurgitation. Heart 2000; 84:606–614.

22. Espinola-Zavaleta N, Gómez-Núñez N, Chávez PY, Sahagun-Sánchez G, Keirns C, Casanova JM, Romero-Cárdenas A, Roldán FJ, Vargas-Barrón J. Evaluation of the response to pharmacological stress in chronic aortic regurgitation. Echocardiography 2001; 18:491–496.

23. Hecker SL, Zabalgoitia M, Ashline P, Oneschuk L, O'Rourke RA, Herrera CJ. Comparison of exercise and dobutamine stress echocardiography in assessing mitral stenosis. Am J Cardiol 1997; 80:1374–1377.

24. Schwammenthal E, Vered Z, Agranat O, Kaplinsky E, Rabinowitz B, Feinberg MS. Impact of atrioventricular compliance on pulmonary artery pressure in mitral stenosis: an exercise echocardiographic study. Circulation 2000; 102:2378–2384.

25. Reis G, Motta MS, Barbosa MM, Esteves WA, Souza SF, Bocchi EA. Dobutamine stress echocardiography for noninvasive assessment and risk stratification of patients with rheumatic mitral stenosis. J Am Coll Cardiol 2004; 43:393–401.

26. Tischler MD, Battle RW, Saha M, Niggel J, LeWinter MM. Observations suggesting a high incidence of exercise-induced severe mitral regurgitation in patients with mild rheumatic mitral valve disease at rest. J Am Coll Cardiol 1995; 25:128–133.

27. Pierard LA, Lancellotti P. The role of ischemic mitral regurgitation in the pathogenesis of acute pulmonary edema. N Engl J Med 2004; 351:1627–1634.

28. Bettadapur MS, Griffin BP, Asher CR. Caring for patients with prosthetic heart valves. Cleve Clin J Med 2002; 69:75–87.

29. Shigenobu M, Sano S. Evaluation of St. Jude Medical mitral valve function by exercise Doppler echocardiography. J Card Surg 1995; 10:161–168.

30. van den Brink RB, Verheul HA, Visser CA, Koelemay MJ, Dunning AJ. Value of exercise Doppler echocardiography in patients with prosthetic or bioprosthetic cardiac valves. Am J Cardiol 1992; 69:367–372.

31. Wu WC, Ireland LA, Sadaniantz A. Evaluation of aortic valve disorders using stress echocardiography. Echocardiography 2004; 21:459–466.

32. Wiseth R, Levang O, Tangen G, Rein KA, Skjaerpe T. Exercise hemodynamics in small (<21-mm) aortic valve prostheses assessed by Doppler echocardiography. Am Heart J 1993; 15:138–146.

33. Tatineni S, Barner HB, Pearson AC, et al. Rest and exercise evaluation of St. Jude Medical and Medtronic Hall prostheses: influence of primary lesion, valvular type, valvular size, and left ventricular function. Circulation 1989; 80:I16–I23.

34. Dressler F, Labovitz A. Exercise evaluation of prosthetic heart valves by Doppler echocardiography: comparison with catheterization studies. Echocardiography 1992; 9:235–241.

35. Bacassis P, Hayot M, Frapier J-M, et al. Postoperative exercise tolerance after aortic valve replacement by small-size prosthesis. J Am Coll Cardiol 2000; 36:871–877.

36. Pibarot P, Dumesnil JG. Prosthesis-patient mismatch: definition, clinical impact, and prevention. Heart 2006; 92:1022–1029.

37. Medalion B, Blackstone E, Lytle B, White J, Arnold J, Cosgrove D. Aortic valve replacement: is valve size important? J Thorac Cardiovasc Surg 2000; 119:963–974.

38. Rahimtoola SH. Is severe valve prosthesis-patient mismatch (VP-PM) associated with a higher mortality? Eur J Cardiothorac Surg 2006; 30:1–3.

39. Blais C, Dumesnil JG, Baillot R, Simard S, Doyle D, Pibarot P. Impact of valve prosthesis-patient mismatch on short-term mortality after aortic valve replacement. Circulation 2003; 108: 983–988.

40. Milano AD, De Carlo M, Mecozzi G, D'Alfonso A, Scioti G, Nardi C, Bortolotti U. Clinical outcome in patients with 19-mm and 21-mm St. Jude aortic prostheses: comparison at long-term follow-up. Ann Thorac Surg 2002; 73:37–43.

41. Picano E, Pálinkás A, Amyot R. Diagnosis of myocardial ischemia in hypertensive patients. J Hypertens 2001; 19: 1177–1183 [Review].

42. Patsilinakos SP, Kranidis AI, Antonelis IP, Filippatos G, Houssianakou IK, Zamanis NI, Sioras E, Tsiotika T, Kardaras F, Anthopoulos LP. Detection of coronary artery disease in patients with severe aortic stenosis with noninvasive methods. Angiology 1999; 50:309–317.

43. Marcus ML, Doty DB, Hiratzka LF, Wright CB, Eastham CL. Decreased coronary reserve: a mechanism for angina pectoris in patients with aortic stenosis and normal coronary arteries. N Engl J Med 1982; 307:1362–1366.

44. Rajappan K, Rimoldi OE, Dutka DP, Ariff B, Pennell DJ, Sheridan DJ, Camici PG. Mechanisms of coronary microcirculatory dysfunction in patients with aortic stenosis and angiographically normal coronary arteries. Circulation 2002; 105:470–476.

45. Bakhtiary F, Schiemann M, Dzemali O, Dogan S, Schächinger V, Ackermann H, Moritz A, Kleine P. Impact of patient-prosthesis mismatch and aortic valve design on coronary flow reserve after aortic valve replacement. J Am Coll Cardiol 2007; 49:790–796.

46. Hildick-Smith DJ, Shapiro LM. Coronary flow reserve improves after aortic valve replacement for aortic stenosis: an adenosine transthoracic echocardiography study. J Am Coll Cardiol 2000; 36:1889–1896.

47. Rigo F. Coronary flow reserve in stress-echo lab: from pathophysiologic toy to diagnostic tool. Cardiovasc Ultrasound 2005 March 25; 3:8.

48. Picano E. Sustainability of medical imaging: education and Debate. BMJ 2004; 328:578–580.

Chapter 6
Valve Substitutes

John Chambers

Introduction

The first clinical valve implantation was of a Starr–Edwards valve in 1960 (Table 6.1). More than 10,000 valves are now imp-lanted each year in the UK, and about 80,000 in the USA. This chapter will describe a classification of valve types, their hemodynamic and clinical assessment, the diagnosis of obstruction and of regurgitation and the management of complications.

Classification

Replacement valves are divided broadly into mechanical and biological valves [1]. An important new category of endovascular valves is now emerging [2] (Table 6.2).

Mechanical Valves

The proportion of mechanical valves implanted in the West is falling and is now below 50%. The main reason is that calcific degenerative aortic valve disease is increasingly common as the population ages and most patients aged over 65

M.Y. Henein (eds.), *Valvular Heart Disease in Clinical Practice*, 241
DOI 10.1007/978-1-84800-275-3_6,
© Springer-Verlag London Limited 2009

TABLE 6.1. Sketch history of replacement heart valves

1902	Brunton: cadaver mitral valvotomy
1908	Cushing and Branch: first mitral valvotomy (in a dog)
1914	Tuffier: first digital dilatation of aortic stenosis
1923	Cutler and Levine: first digital dilatation of mitral stenosis
1948	Harken/Bailey/Brock: closed mitral valvotomy
1949	Templeton and Gibbon: mitral reconstruction
1952	Hufnagel: caged ball valve
1953	Gibbon: introduction of bypass machine
1956	Murray: homograft valve for aortic and mitral use
1960	Harken: first caged ball valve. Starr: first clinical Starr–Edwards valve implanted
1965	Binet: first aortic heterograft
1968	Hancock, Carpentier: first glutaraldehyde and formaldehyde stented heterografts
1969	Bjork: first tilting disc valve
1970	Ionescu: stented bovine pericardial valve
1977	St Jude Medical: first bileaflet mechanical valve
1980	St Jude Medical Toronto stentless valve

will receive a biological valve. In addition, mitral repair rates are rising so that fewer mechanical replacement valves are implanted. The most frequently implanted mechanical valve is the bileaflet which is the least obstructive design. The various bileaflet designs differ in the composition and purity of the pyrolytic carbon, in the shape and opening angle of the leaflets, the design of the pivots, the size and shape of the housing and the design of the sewing ring, e.g., the St Jude Medical valve has a deep housing with pivots contained on flanges, the Carbomedics has a shorter housing allowing the leaflet tips to be imaged clearly on echocardiography and the MCRI On-X valve has a long, flared housing.

Biological Valves

The most frequently implanted biological replacement valve is the stented xenografts. The stent is a plastic or wire structure covered in fabric with the cusps of the valve placed inside and a sewing ring attached outside. The valve cusps usually

TABLE 6.2. Designs of replacement heart valve

Biological
Autograft (Ross operation)
Homograft usually aortic, occasionally pulmonary
Stented heterograft, e.g., Hancock (porcine), Mosaic (porcine),
    Baxter Perimount (pericardial), Carpentier–Edwards
    (standard and supra-annular porcine), Intact (porcine), Labcor
    (porcine tricomposite), Biocor (porcine tri-composite),
    Mitroflow (bovine pericardial)
Stentless heterograft, e.g., Toronto (St Jude Medical),
    Cryolife-O'Brien, Freestyle (Medtronic), Baxter Prima, Biocor
    PSB tricomposite, Sorin Pericarbon (pericardial)

Mechanical
Ball-cage, e.g., Starr–Edwards
Single tilting disk, e.g., Bjork–Shiley, Medtronic–Hall, Monostrut,
    Omniscience, Ultracor
Bileaflet, e.g., St Jude Medical, Carbomedics, MCRI On-X, ATS,
    Sorin Bicarbon, Edwards Tekna, Edwards Mira

---

consist of pericardium or a porcine aortic valve. The porcine aortic valve may be used in its entirety as in the Carpentier–Edwards valve, but there is a muscle bar at the base of the right coronary cusp which reduces the orifice available for flow. This cusp may therefore be excised and replaced by a single cusp from another pig or, more frequently, each cusp may be taken from up to three different pigs as in the Medtronic Mosaic or the St Jude Epic or Carbomedics Synergy. Pericardium is cut using a template and sewn inside the stent posts or occasionally, as in the Carbomedics Mitroflow, to the outside. Usually the pericardium is bovine, but sometimes porcine and, occasionally equine or kangaroo.

A stentless heterograft valve usually consists of a preparation of porcine aorta. The aorta may be relatively long (Medtronic Freestyle) or may be sculpted to fit under the coronary arteries (Edwards Toronto, Cryolife-O'Brien). Some are tricomposite and one is made out of bovine pericardium (Sorin Freedom). Most designs are technically hard to implant and require long bypass times which may be a disadvantage in a high-risk patient. The potential advantage is better hemodynamic function, durability and complication rates than for stented valves. There is some evidence to support better hemodynamic function in the least obstructive designs, but no evidence yet of better durability or complication rates. For all these reasons, stentless valves are not commonly implanted.

A homograft is a human aortic valve or, less commonly, pulmonary valve which is usually cryopreserved and left unstented. A homograft has good durability if harvested early after death and does not need anticoagulation and so may be used as an alternative to a mechanical valve in the young. A homograft may also be used for choice in the presence of endocarditis since it allows wide clearance of infection with replacement of the aortic root and valve and the possibility of using the attached flap of donor mitral leaflet to repair perforations in the base of the recipient's anterior mitral leaflet. The disadvantage is that durability may be disappointing when the valve is harvested relatively late after death, particularly when a pulmonary homograft is placed in the aortic position. Reoperation in the presence of a calcified homograft root may be difficult.

The Ross procedure consists of substituting the patient's own pulmonary valve for the diseased aortic valve. Usually a homograft is then implanted in the pulmonary position. The rationale for such a complex procedure is that a living valve with good durability is placed in the important aortic side while the replacement valve is placed in the low pressure right side. The procedure has a relatively high early complication rate but good long-term results. There is evidence that the autograft grows which is particularly important for avoiding repeated surgery in children. It may also be relatively resistant to infection.

Biological valves have the advantage of not needing treatment with warfarin, but the disadvantage of primary failure beginning after about 7 years in the aortic position and 5 years in the mitral position [3]. By contrast, mechanical valves effectively have no primary failure, but need anticoagulation and therefore being open to the possibility of anticoagulant-related hemorrhage. In general, patients needing aortic valve replacement are usually given a biological valve if they are aged more than 65 years and a mechanical valve if they are aged below 60 years [4]. In between 60 and 65 years, the choice depends on individual patient factors including their own preference. Exceptions are the younger person unwilling or unable to take anticoagulants in whom a Ross procedure or homograft are alternatives. In patients not suitable for mitral valve repair, a mechanical valve is usually implanted below the age of 65 years and a biological valve above the age of 70 years. Individual factors must again be applied in the range 65–70 years. Improvements in life-expectancy mean that many patients with biological valves are beginning to live long enough to require consideration of redo surgery.

Some specific situations are outside these general rules. Some surgeons preferentially use a biological valve in a woman considering child-birth to avoid the need for warfarin [5]. However, this necessitates further surgery after a short duration long enough to complete the family. The relative merits of mechanical and biological valves remain unresolved. Recent attempts to combine all events including anticoagulant-related hemorrhage suggest that survival free of re-do surgery or adverse events may be similar for both types of valve [6, 7]. The choice of valve is made particularly difficult because durability data on the newer designs including the stentless valves is lacking. It is important to individualize the choice of valve and to involve patients in that choice if they want to be.

Assessment

Echocardiography is the mainstay of assessment [8]. Fluoroscopy or CT scanning may still be useful for the imaging of leaflets if obstruction is suspected. A study should be performed in the early postoperative period to act as a baseline. Every valve is different and this study acts as a 'finger-print' against which to compare future studies. The timing of the baseline study depends on circumstances. Ideally, it should be at the first postoperative visit usually after 4–6 weeks when the chest wound has healed, chest wall edema has resolved and left ventricular function has recovered. However, if the patient is being transferred and may not return, it may be best to perform the study before hospital discharge. The echocardiography of replacement heart valves is more demanding than of native valves for the following reasons:

- Obstruction. Almost all replacement valves are obstructive compared to normal native valves. The differentiation between normal and pathological obstruction may be difficult
- Regurgitation. Transprosthetic regurgitation is normal for almost all mechanical valves and for many biological valves. This can be mistaken for pathological regurgitation.
- Normal variability. The appearance, forward-flow and patterns of regurgitation differ between valve designs. Experience gained from one valve type may lead to confusion if extrapolated to another.
- Technical difficulties. Shielding from the ultrasound beam by mechanical parts can obscure vegetations or a regurgitant jet. Blooming or reverberation artifacts can cause overdiagnosis of abnormal masses or of calcification.

Appearance

A replacement valve usually consists of cusps or an occluder (tilting disc or mechanical leaflet) inside a valve housing and attached to a sewing ring. These structures are usually visible on transthoracic echocardiography and are more obvious in the mitral position. For a valve in the aortic position it may be difficult to image a cage which is usually seen best in an apical long-axis view. There should be no abnormal extrinsic masses attached to the valve although stitches may be seen and thin fibrinous strands are normal. It is normal to see echoes resembling bubbles in the left ventricle in the presence of a replacement mitral valve (Figure 6.1). These

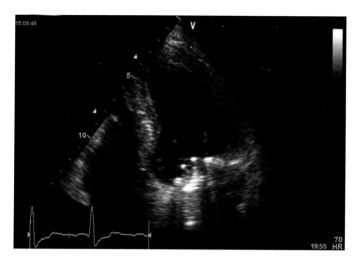

FIGURE 6.1. Microcavitations from a bileaflet mechanical mitral valve. These are normal and almost certainly have no pathological significance.

occur with all designs but are most frequent with bileaflet mechanical valves. Their origin is not known. They are probably benign although occasional reports link them to abnormalities of higher cognitive function. Stentless valves may be surrounded by edema and hematoma Figure 6.6. This ultimately resolves over 3–6 months and is associated with a rise in effective orifice area and a fall in transaortic pressure difference. On transesophageal echocardiography, the appearance may be impossible to differentiate from an abscess.

Rocking of the valve suggests dehiscence and is proved by overlaying color Doppler and demonstrating a paraprosthetic regurgitant jet. Usually, rocking in the aortic position implies a large dehiscence, about 40% of the sewing ring. In the mitral position, if the surgeon has retained the posterior leaflet there may be rocking without dehiscence.

If the valve is biological the cusps should be thin (around 1 mm) and fully mobile with no extraneous masses. There should be no movement of any part of the cusp behind the plane of the annulus. If the valve is mechanical, the occluder should open quickly and fully. The color map should fill the whole orifice in all views.

Forward Flow

Measurements should be taken over one to three cycles in sinus rhythm but usually five in atrial fibrillation. Measurements needed in the aortic position are peak velocity; derived mean and peak pressure difference and effective orifice area by the continuity equation. In the mitral position, measurements needed are peak velocity, mean pressure difference and pressure half-time. In the tricuspid position, measurements needed are peak velocity, mean pressure difference and pressure half-time.

High flow can cause unrepresentatively high peak velocities in replacement aortic valves. It is important to derive the mean pressure difference because it is calculated using the whole wave-form and better reflects function than using the peak velocity alone. In a normal valve, the subaortic velocity may not be negligible compared with the transaortic velocity so the long form of the modified Bernoulli equation should be used. Peak pressure drop across the aortic valve is calculated from the formula:

Peak $\triangle P = 4(v_2^2 - v_1^2)$, where v_1 and v_2 are peak velocities in the subaortic and transaortic signal, respectively. Mean pressure difference cannot be derived from the respective mean velocities. It should ideally be derived from multiple calculations of pressure difference using instantaneous velocities on the pulsed and continuous wave forms. This can be estimated from the online software as aortic mean ΔP–subaortic mean ΔP.

Because of the flow dependency of velocity and pressure difference, effective area by the continuity equation (EOA) should be calculated routinely from the formula:

$EOA = CSA \times VTI_1/VTI_2$, where CSA is left ventricular outflow cross-sectional area in cm^2 calculated from the diameter assuming circular cross-section; VTI_1 is subaortic velocity time integral in cm and VTI_2 is aortic velocity time integral in cm. Errors arise if the peak velocity is used in place of the velocity integral. It is not usually appropriate to substitute the labeled size of the replacement valve for the left ventricular outflow tract diameter because this may differ widely from its true size [9]. For serial studies, it is reasonable to use the ratio of the velocity integrals since this avoids measuring the left ventricular outflow tract diameter.

For the mitral valve, the subvalve velocity is negligible and in any case cannot be measured. The formula Peak $\triangle P = 4(v_2^2)$ can therefore be used and the mean pressure difference taken from the continuous wave signal. It is not appropriate to use the Hatle formula to estimate orifice area. This is only valid for moderate or severe stenosis with orifice area <1.5 cm^2. For valve areas above this, the pressure half-time mainly reflects atrial and left ventricular compliance characteristics and loading conditions.

Few tricuspid replacement valves are implanted, but the same methods are applied as for the mitral position. The pressure half-time is even more variable on the right than on the left side of the heart. For a valve in any position, forward-flow velocities and derived pressure differences (gradient) cannot be interpreted without knowing the valve type and size.

Regurgitation

Minor regurgitation is normal in virtually all mechanical valves. Early valves had a closing volume as the leaflet closed followed by true regurgitation around the occluder. For the Starr–Edwards, there is a small closing volume and usually little or no true regurgitation. The single tilting disk valves have both types of regurgitation, but the pattern may vary. The Bjork–Shiley valve has a minor and major jet from the two orifices while the Medtronic–Hall valve has a single large jet through a central hole in the disk. The bileaflet valves have continuous leakage through the pivotal points where the lugs of the leaflets are held in the housing. These are thought to prevent the formation of thrombus at sites of stasis and are called 'washing jets'. The associated regurgitant fraction is directly related to the size of the valve and is also larger at low cardiac outputs. Although the regurgitant fraction is usually no larger than 10–15%, the associated color jet can look large, up to 5 cm long and 1 cm wide. They are usually found in formation, two from each pivotal point giving a characteristic appearance on imaging in a plane just below the valve. Sometimes, these single pivotal washing jets divide into two or three separate 'plumes' and in some valve designs such as the St Jude Medical there may be a jet around the edge of one or other leaflet. The jets are invariably low in momentum so that they are homogenous in color with aliasing confined to the base of the jet.

Regurgitation through the valve is also increasingly reported in normal biological valves. This is mainly because echocardiography machines are becoming increasingly sensitive. Stentless valves including homografts and autografts are more likely than the stented valves to have minor regurgitant jets, usually at the point of apposition of all three cusps or at one or more commissures. In stented valves, the regurgitation is usually at the point of apposition of the cusps.

Diagnosis of Obstruction

Mitral Position

Heavily calcified cusps and reduced occluder motion are the most reliable signs of obstruction, particularly for valves in the mitral position since the cusps or occluder are usually imaged easily. In a bileaflet mechanical valve, partial obstruction may be obvious when one leaflet moves less than the other (Figure 6.2). Even if image quality is suboptimal, color mapping can identify obstruction by showing a narrowed, high-velocity inflow jet with 'wrap-around' aliasing although transesophageal imaging may often be necessary to confirm this. In a stenotic stented biological valve, the jet can be

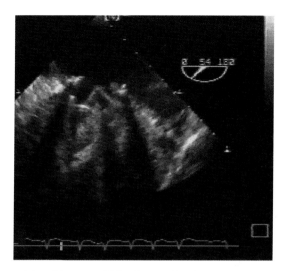

FIGURE 6.2.   Obstructed bileaflet mechanical mitral valve. This is a diastolic frame and the lateral leaflet is held in the closed position within a mass of thrombus.

narrow at the level of the immobile cusps, but can expand rapidly to fill the orifice toward the tips of the stents. It is therefore easy to miss the abnormality. Severe impairment of left ventricular function may also cause reduced valve opening but this will be associated with a thin, low-velocity inflow signal on color mapping.

Quantitative Doppler confirms the diagnosis if the pressure half-time is markedly prolonged usually to >200 ms with an elevated peak velocity usually >2.0 m/s and mean pressure difference >10 mmHg. Indirect signs, including a rise in pulmonary artery pressure or a slow-filling left ventricle may occasionally help.

TEE is often necessary to confirm the diagnosis of obstruction and always to determine the cause, notably thrombosis and pannus (see complications).

Aortic Position

High transaortic velocities are common in normally functioning aortic replacement valves, particularly of label size 19 or 21. Most are caused by patient-prosthesis mismatch which must be distinguished from pathological obstruction. Patient-prosthesis mismatch occurs when an implanted valve is too small for the size of the patient and is defined by an EOA indexed to BSA of <0.85 cm^2/m^2. Severe patient-prosthesis mismatch is defined by an EOAi <0.65 cm^2/m^2. The differentiation is made as shown in Table 6.3 and relies on comparison with normal ranges for that design and size [10, 11] and imaging the leaflets. If the cusps or occluder are not well seen transthoracically it is necessary to perform transesophageal imaging or consider fluoroscopy or CT scanning [12].

Pressure recovery is one cause of a discrepancy in the pressure difference estimated between cardiac catheterization and Doppler ultrasound. As flow lines diverge downstream from the orifice of the valve, kinetic energy falls and static pressure rises. The pressure difference is therefore maximal where the hemodynamic orifice is smallest at the vena contracta and rises downstream from this point. Doppler ultrasound estimates pressure difference at the vena contracta, but cardiac catheterization measures the difference between the LV and a point downstream from the orifice

TABLE 6.3. High velocities: differentiating patient-prosthesis mismatch from pathological obstruction

	Patient prosthesis mismatch	Pathological obstruction
EOAi	In normal range for design and size	Lower than normal range
Change with time	Same as baseline after surgery	Fall over serial studies
Cusp or occluder	Normal appearance and movement	Reduced motion

beyond whip artifact where the pressure will have recovered. Pressure recovery is usually complete about 10 orifice diameters beyond the valve. The degree of pressure recovered will be reduced if significant energy is lost from turbulence and will be relatively great if the aortic root is small. Some biological valves which open well act hemodynamically as funnels allowing flow lines to stay attached without causing pressure recovery. There is an additional source of pressure recovery between the leaflets of bileaflet mechanical valves. Pressure recovery is not a clinical problem unless the results of cardiac catheterization & Doppler are compared which should not usually be necessary. The effect of pressure recovery is accommodated in published normal ranges.

Tricuspid Position

These valves are not commonly implanted. Obstruction is suggested by reduced cusp or occluder motion or a narrowed color signal. An engorged, unreactive inferior vena cava with a dilated right atrium and small right ventricle all suggest tricuspid obstruction. A transtricuspid peak velocity >1.5 m/s in the absence of significant tricuspid regurgitation or a mean pressure difference >5 mmHg is also suggestive [13]. The pressure half-time is variable and not helpful unless markedly prolonged to >250 ms.

Diagnosis of Regurgitation

Is it Pathological?

Many valves have transprosthetic regurgitation as a normal finding or even a design feature. However, in a biological valve, a broad jet, particularly if it is bigger than on previous studies, is a sign of primary failure or endocarditis. Large transprosthetic jets are uncommon in mechanical valves, but can occur if the leaflet is held open by thrombus or a vegetation.

Paraprosthetic leaks have their origin outside the sewing ring and can usually be detected transthoracically even in the mitral position. Although the mechanical parts of the valve shield the interatrial part of the jet from ultrasound, a significant jet has a neck and an intraventricular portion of flow acceleration. Even these are occasionally invisible for posterior paraprosthetic mitral regurgitation. However, the majority of paraprosthetic leaks occur at the mitral-aortic fibrosa. It may sometimes be difficult to differentiate a paraprosthetic jet from an asymmetric jet through the valve especially those beginning at the base of cusps or at a commissure and TEE is then indicated (**Figure** 6.3).

Paraprosthetic leaks are pathological by definition but may not be of clinical significance. Small paraprosthetic leaks are more common in valves with thin sewing rings or patients with poor tissue, e.g., as a result of endocarditis or Marfan syndrome.

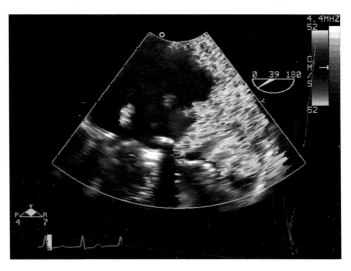

FIGURE 6.3. Paraprosthetic mitral regurgitation. There is a broad jet originating just outside the sewing ring. The small, low momentum pivotal washing jets can also be seen within the orifice.

Quantification

Broadly, the same methods can be used as for native regurgitation. However, assessing the height of an aortic jet relative to the left ventricular outflow tract diameter may be difficult if it is eccentric and care must be taken to measure the diameter of the jet perpendicular to its axis. Multiple small normal transprosthetic jets cannot be quantified accurately, but this is not necessary in clinical practice. For paraprosthetic jets, the proportion of the circumference of the sewing ring occupied by the jet gives an approximate guide to severity: mild (<10%), moderate (10–25%), severe (>25%).

Because of shielding it may be difficult to quantify a jet in the mitral position. Although TEE is usually necessary, the likelihood of severe regurgitation can be judged by indirect signs predominantly overactivity of the left ventricle or occasionally a rise in pulmonary artery pressure compared with an earlier study. A dense continuous wave regurgitant signal is another useful transthoracic sign, particularly if it depressurizes rapidly. When associated with a low systolic LV and systemic pressure, this signal resembles that obtained from aortic stenosis, an error all the easier to make if the neck of the paraprosthetic jet is at the mitral-aortic fibrosa and the interatrial portion runs parallel with the aorta.

Complications

There is no ideal replacement valve and all can have complications [14]:

- Primary failure
- Thrombosis
- Mechanical obstruction by pannus
- Thromboembolism
- Endocarditis
- Dehiscence
- Hemolysis
- Hemorrhage

Primary failure means deterioration of the valve without secondary infection or other cause. It is almost exclusively a problem of the biological valves and occurs more quickly for the mitral than the aortic position. The survival to 10 years is about 70% in the aortic and 60% in the mitral position. Durability is worse in the younger patient (aged under 60 years for the aortic and under 65 years for the mitral position). It may also be affected by blood pressure and cholesterol levels. Leaflet escape has occurred for a small number of types of mechanical valve notably the Bjork–Shiley Convexo–Concave.

Thrombosis is relatively uncommon in biological valves and in mechanical valves in the aortic position (Figure 6.2). It occurs at a rate of about 0.1–0.2% p.a. in mechanical valve in the mitral position and more frequently in the tricuspid position [3]. Thrombolysis is the treatment of choice for right-sided thrombosis while surgery is the treatment of choice for left-sided thrombosis. Thrombolysis can be considered for left-sided thrombosis if the patient is critically ill but no cardiac surgery is available or if the patient has significant comorbidity.

Pannus is overgrowth of endothelium which extends over the orifice (Figure 6.4) and may cause obstruction directly or indirectly by interfering with the opening of the occluder. It is mainly a problem of mechanical valves and may occasionally hold an occluder open to cause regurgitation. It may also induce secondary thrombosis or thromboembolism occasionally making the differentiation between pannus and thrombus difficult (Table 6.4). Thrombus usually causes relatively low density echoes which are often continuous with a mass outside the valve, particularly in the atrial appendage. Pannus is typically highly echogenic and may be difficult to distinguish from the sewing ring. The valve may look normal at first but with an abnormally small orifice diameter. It is usually imaged on echocardiography (Figure 6.4), but if image quality is inadequate may be seen on CT scanning [15]. Pannus is treated by redo surgery.

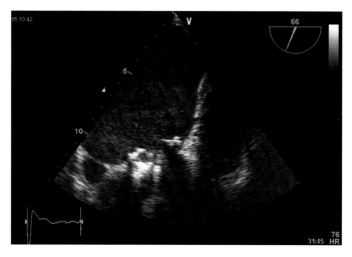

FIGURE 6.4.   Pannus. There is a thin highly echogenic line extending from the sewing ring over the orifice.

Thromboembolism is related to patient factors such as age and cardiac rhythm as well as to the position of the replacement valve. It occurs at a rate of 1–4% p.a. in mechanical and 1–2% p.a. in biological valves and is more common for valves in the mitral than the aortic position. ESC guidelines [16] recommend full investigation of all thromboembolic events (CT

TABLE 6.4.   Differentiation of thrombus and pannus

	Favors pannus	Favors thrombosis
Duration of symptoms	Long (maybe several months)	Acute
Timing	>6 months after surgery	Early
INR	Therapeutic	Subtherapeutic
TEE appearance	Highly echogenic	Plump relatively low density

scan of the brain, carotid studies) since the replacement valve cannot be assumed to be the origin.

Endocarditis occurs in approximately 3% of patients in the first year then about 0.5–1% per year thereafter. It is similar in frequency in mechanical and biological valves. The stentless valves (autograft, homograft and stentless heterografts) are perceived to be relatively resistant to infection although this remains unproved. Vegetations and local complications (dehiscence, abscess, perforation, fistula) may be obvious even on transthoracic echocardiography especially if the valve is biological. However, if the valve is mechanical, vegetations are often difficult to detect transthoracically and TEE is then necessary (Figure 6.5).

The echocardiogram must never be interpreted outside the clinical context. It is possible to differentiate neither vegetations from a segment of disrupted cusp nor generalized valve thickening as a result of infection from primary failure even

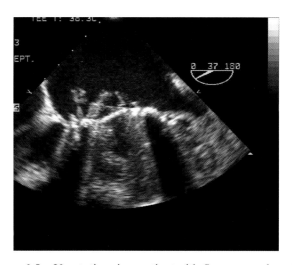

FIGURE 6.5.   Vegetations in a patient with *S. aureus* endocarditis. The transthoracic study was normal despite the fact that the TEE showed a large mass of vegetations encircling the whole sewing ring.

on TEE. Similarly, normal swelling and hematoma around a recently implanted stentless valve can not be differentiated from an abscess (Figure 6.6).

Prosthetic endocarditis is more likely to require surgery than for native endocarditis. Surgery is usually necessary

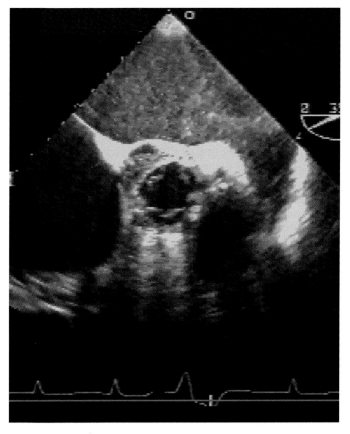

FIGURE 6.6. 'Pseudoabscess'. Thickening of the aortic root as a result of hematoma and edema is normal in the first few months after implantation of a stentless aortic valve. This is not distinguishable on echocardiography from an abscess.

for early endocarditis, particularly involving *Staphylococcus aureus* or fungi. It is also necessary if there is significant prosthetic dysfunction or complications such as abscess formation [17, 18].

Dehiscence is the opening of a gap outside the sewing ring leading to paraprosthetic regurgitation. This may occur at the time of surgery as a result of technical error or poor tissues as a result of heavy calcification, endocarditis or abnormalities of collagen, e.g., in Marfan syndrome. It is more likely in valves with relatively thin sewing rings and less likely in valves with bulky sewing rings (e.g., Starr–Edwards). It may occur late as a result of endocarditis, but also on occasions with disintegration of the sewing ring and degeneration of the patient annulus.

Mild hemolysis occurs in almost all mechanical valves, but is usually compensated. The blood lactate dehydrogenase and bilirubin levels are high and the haptoglobin level low, but the hemoglobin level normal. Anemia occasionally occurs in the presence of an aggravating cause such as iron deficiency, but otherwise suggests the presence of a paraprosthetic leak. This is often small and clinically occult. It may only be detected by TEE.

Bleeding Guideline INR targets depend on the type of valve and the presence of non-prosthetic thromboembolic risk factors (Table 6.5) [16] which are the presence of atrial fibrillation, a left atrial diameter >50 mm, LV ejection fraction < 35%, the presence of a mechanical valve in any position other than the aortic. The thromboembolic risk for a valve cannot be assumed from its design and has to be judged by clinical data. Thus the Medtronic–Hall valve is classed as low-risk, the Bjork–Shiley as medium risk and the Omniscience as high risk although all are tilting disk valves.

The management of a high INR depends on whether there is bleeding. In the absence of bleeding, ESC guidelines recommend admission if the INR is ≥6 with the withdrawal of warfarin. It is vital to avoid giving vitamin K which risks valve thrombosis. If the INR is ≥10, the use of FFP can be considered. If there is bleeding and it cannot be controlled by

TABLE 6.5. Target INR levels [16, 20]

Thromboembolic risk	No risk factors[a]	Risk factors[a]
Low[b]	2.5	3.0
Medium[c]	3.0	3.5
High[d]	3.5	4.0

[a] The risk factors are atrial fibrillation, left atrium >50 mm, LV ejection fraction <35%, valve in the mitral, tricuspid or pulmonary position

[b] Medtronic–Hall, St Jude Medical, Carbomedics

[c] Bjork–Shiley, generic bileaflet mechanical

[d] Starr–Edwards, Omniscience.

local pressure, factor VII or FFP should be given. Vitamin K can be considered if the bleeding is critically dangerous, e.g., intracerebral. Bleeding is included as a valve-related complication because warfarin is essential for mechanical valves and so cannot be dissociated from the valve itself. It occurs at a rate of about 2% p.a. in mechanical valves, 1% p.a. for biological mitral valves and 0.5% p.a. for biological aortic valves. Bleeding and thromboembolism rates are reduced by self-monitoring of anticoagulation [19].

Conclusions

Echocardiography of replacement heart valves is more demanding than for native valves. There are some key points:

- Quantitative Doppler should always be interpreted in the clinical context; normal ranges vary with design, position and size
- Velocities are flow-dependent; always calculate effective orifice area for valves in the aortic position
- Do not use valve size in place of left ventricular outflow tract diameter in calculating the effective orifice area
- The pressure half-time method for calculating effective orifice area is not valid in normal replacement mitral valves

- Transvalvar regurgitation is normal in almost all mechanical valves and many biological valves
- Transthoracic and transesophageal echocardiography are complimentary and should not be considered in isolation

References

1. Jamieson WRE. Effective current and advanced prostheses for cardiac valvular replacement and reconstructive surgery. Surgical Technology International 2002.
2. Gruse E, Schuler G, Bhellsfeld L et al. Percutanems aortic valve replacement for severe aortic stenosis in high-risk patients using the second- and current third-generation self-expanding. Corevalve prosthesis: device success and 30-day clinical outcome. JACC 2007; 50:69–76.
3. Grunkemeier GL, Li H-H, Naftel DC, Starr A, Rahimtoola SH. Long-term performance of heart valve prostheses. Curr Probl Cardiol 2000; 25:73–156.
4. Rahimtoola S. Choice of prosthetic heart valve for adult patients. JACC 2003; 41:893–904.
5. Elkayam U, Bitar F. Valvular heart disease and pregnancy: Part II Prosthetic valves. JACC 2005; 46:403–410.
6. Khan SS, Trento A, DeRbertis M, et al. Twenty-year comparison of tissue and mechanical valve replacement. J Thorac Cardiovasc Surg 2001; 122:257–259.
7. Puvimanasinghe JPA, Takkenberg JJM, Edwards MB, et al. Comparison of outcomes after valve replacement with a mechanical valve or a bioprosthesis using microsimulation. Heart 2004; 90:1172–1178.
8. Chambers J, Fraser A, Lawford P, Nihoyannopoulos P, Simpson I. Echocardiographic assessment of artificial heart valves: British Society of echocardiography position paper. British Heart J 1994; 71(Suppl 4):6–14.
9. Cochran RP, Kunzelman KS. Discrepancies between labelled and actual dimensions of prosthetic valves and sizers. J Card Surg 1996; 11:318–324.
10. Rosenhek R, Binder T, Maurer G, Baumgartner H. Normal values for Doppler echocardiographic assessment of heart valve prostheses. J Am Coll Cardiol 2003; 16:1116–1127.

11. Rajani R, Mukherjee D, Chambers J. Doppler echocardiography in normally functioning replacement aortic valves: a review of 129 studies. J Heart Valve Dis 2007; 16:519–535.

12. Leborgne L, Renard C, Tribouilloy C. Usefulness of ECG-gated multi-detector computed tomography for the diagnosis of prosthetic valve dysfunction. Europ Heart J 2006; 2537.

13. Connolly HM, Miller FA, Taylor CL, Naessens JM, Seward JB, Tajik AJ. Doppler hemodynamic profiles of 82 clinically and echocardiographically normal tricuspid valve prostheses. Circulation 1993; 88:2722–2727.

14. Edmunds LH, Clark RE, Cohn LH, Grunkemeier GL, Miller DC, Weisel RD. Guidelines for reporting morbidity and mortality after cardiac valvular operations. J Thorac Cardiovasc Surg 1996; 112:708–711.

15. Teshima, H, Hayashiba N, Enomoto N, Aoyaci S, Okmon K, Uchida M. Detection of pannus by multidetector-row computed tomocremay. Ann. Thorm Sury 2003; 75:1631–1633.

16. Vahanian A, Baumgartner H, Bax J, et al. Guidelines on the management of valvular heart disease. Europ Heart J 2007; 28:230–268.

17. Habib G, Tribouilloy C, Thuny F, et al. Prosthetic valve endocarditis: who will need surgery? A multicentre study of 104 cases. Heart 2005; 91:954–959.

18. Akowuah EF, Davies W, Oliver S, Stephens J, Riaz I, Zadik P, Cooper G. Prosthetic valve endocarditis: early and late outcome following medical or surgical treatment. Heart 2003; 89:29–72.

19. Heneghan C, Alonso-Coello P, Garcia-Alamino JM, Perera R, Meats E, Glasziou P. Self-monitoring of oral anticoagulation: a systematic review and meta-analysis. Brit Med J 2006; 367: 404–411.

20. Butchart EG, Gohlke-Barwolf C, Antunes MJ, et al. Recommendations for the management of patients after heart valve surgery. Europ Heart J 2005; 26:2463–2471.

Chapter 7
Native and Prosthetic Valve Endocarditis

Maurizio Galderisi and Sergio Mondillo

Infective endocarditis is a cardiac infection that involves valve leaflets, endocardium, chordae tendinae, congenital defects and anastomosis sites. It may also affect artificial intracardiac materials including artificial valves, conduits, catheters, shunt occluders and assist devices. The characteristic lesion of infective endocarditis is the *vegetation* which is made of aggregate of infective organisms, inflammatory cells and blood platelets and could take various shapes and sizes.

Classification of Endocarditis

Infective endocarditis is usually classified according to its localization on native valves and on prosthetic valves.

1. *Native valve endocarditis* (NVE): Endocarditis of the native valves usually has a substrate for infection in 55–75% of cases. Mitral valve prolapse represents the highest predisposing valve lesion (10 times greater than normal valves) and accounts for up to 25% of overall incidence of NVE cases. Another risk for NVE is through i.v. lines, particularly on the tricuspid valve. NVE can be either acute, commonly caused by *Staphylococcus aureus* or subacute which is caused by HACEK group including *Haemophilus, Actinobacillus, Cardiobacterium, Eikenella* and *Kingella*.

M.Y. Henein (ed.), *Valvular Heart Disease in Clinical Practice*,
DOI 10.1007/978-1-84800-275-3_7,
© Springer-Verlag London Limited 2009

2. *Prosthetic valve endocarditis* (PVE): Endocarditis of the prosthetic valves accounts for up to 30% of all cases of IE. *S. aureus* is the commonest causing organism. While early PVE (<60 days) after cardiac surgery is commonly caused by *Staphylococcus epidermidis, S. aureus*, gram-negative microorganisms or *Candida,* late PVE is caused by *Streptococcus*, *S. aureus or* HACEK group. PVE starts at the interface between the prosthesis and the annulus then it extends toward the prosthetic cusps, or the tissue valve leaflets. Furthermore, the infection may spread to the structures adjacent to the annulus, e.g., the sinusus or the native mitral valve leaflets themselves in the case of aortic valve endocarditis.

Diagnosis of Infective Endocarditis

Diagnosis of endocarditis is usually made clinically and confirmed by echocardiography. Signs and symptoms of infective endocarditis are included in the major and minor criteria of the Duke University [1] (Table 7.1). Echocardiography is the best technique for non-invasive visualization of vegetations and abscess formation [2] (Tables 7.2 and 7.3).

Native Valve Endocarditis (NVE)

Transthoracic echocardiography (TTE) can detect vegetations on left and right heart valves [3], Figure 7.1. In left-sided NVE, vegetation size, consistency and extent of mobility have all been found to predict complications. In multivariate analysis, vegetation size, extent of mobility have emerged as the two optimal predictors of complications with 70% sensitivity and 92% specificity for mitral valve endocarditis and 76% sensitivity and 62% specificity for aortic valve endocarditis [4]. Harmonic imaging has significantly improved the accuracy of TTE in detecting the presence of native valve vegetations. It provides better visualization of low-level signals

TABLE 7.1. Duke criteria for infective endocarditis

I. Definite infective endocarditis

Pathologic criteria: Microorganisms demonstrated by culture or histology in a vegetation or in intracardiac abscess

Pathologic lesions: Vegetation or intracardiac abscess confirmed by histology

II. Possible infective endocarditis

Findings consistent with but failing short of I

Definite but not III

Rejected

III. Rejected

Firm alternative diagnosis for manifestations

Resolution of manifestations with 4 days or less of antibiotics

No surgical or pathologic evidence with 4 days or less of antibiotics

Major criteria

1. Positive blood culture for IE:

Clinical criteria: Two major criteria or one major and three minor criteria or five minor criteria

Minor criteria

1. Predisposing heart condition or intravenous drug history.

TABLE 7.1. Continued.

Typical microorganisms for IE from two separate blood cultures in absence of a primary focus or persistently positive blood cultures of an IE consistent organism recovered from cultures drawn at least 12 h apart or the majority of four cultures spanning more than 1 h. Persistently positive blood cultures of an IE

2. Evidence of endocardial involvement: Echo positive for IE (oscillating mass on valve/apparatus or in jet pathway or implanted material in absence of alternative explanation or abscess or new prosthetic dehiscence).

3. New murmur of valve regurgitation (increase or change of pre-existing murmur not sufficient).

2. Fever $\geq$38°C.

3. Vascular phenomena. Major arterial emboli, septic pulmonary embolism/infarction, mycotic aneurysm (with and without hemorrage), conjunctival hemorrage, Janeway lesions.

4. Immunologic phenomena: Glomerulonephritis, Osler's nodes, Roth spots, rheumatoid factor.

5. Microbiologic evidence: Positive blood culture but not meeting major criteria (exclude coagulase-negative staphylococci and organisms not causing IE) or serologic evidence of IE organisms.

6. Echo consistent with but not meeting major criteria for IE.

Modified from Durack DTY, Lukes AS, Bright DE. Am J Ned 1994; 96:200–209.

TABLE 7.2. Indication of TTE for diagnosis of infective endocarditis

Indications	Class
Detection of valvular vegetations with or without positive blood cultures	1 (level b evidence)
Detection of the kind of valvular lesion inducing hemodynamic compromision during IE	1 (level b evidence)
Detection of IE complications	1 (level b evidence)
Diagnostic re-evaluation in patients at high risk (e.g., patients with virulent microorganisms, with clinic worsening, with persistent fewer, new onset murmur, persistent bacteremia)	1 (level c evidence)
Diagnosis of IE on prosthetic valve in presence of persistent fewer, without bacteremia o new onset murmur	2a (level c evidence)
Diagnostic re-evaluation of IE on prosthetic valve during antibiotic therapy, in absence of clinical worsening	2b (level c evidence)
TEE not indicated to re-evaluate forms of IE on native valves not complicated (including absence of regurgitation at basal Doppler echo) during antibiotic therapy, in absence of clinical worsening or persistent fewer	3 (level c evidence)

Modified from Bonow et al., ACC/AHA Practice guidelines, J Am Coll Cardiol 2006; 48:1–148.

arising from the endocardium [3–6]. Transesophageal (TEE) technique has significantly increased the accuracy of echocardiography for diagnosing vegetations, Figures 7.2 and 7.3. A negative TEE has a negative predictive value of 86–97% for diagnosing endocarditis [7]. It is always important to consider TEE findings with respect to disease stage, patients with an

TABLE 7.3. Clinical indications of TEE for diagnosis of infective endocarditis

Indications	Class
Evaluation of valvular lesion in symptomatic patients with IE when TTE is not diagnostic	1 (level c evidence)
Diagnosis of IE in patients with valvular heart disease and positive blood culture, when TTE is not diagnostic	1 (level c evidence)
Diagnosis of complications of IE (abscess, perforation, shunts)	1 (level c evidence)
First-level examination of valvular prosthesis	1 (level c evidence)
Pre-surgery evaluation in patients with known IE, when TTE is not diagnostic or the surgery is not urgent	1 (level c evidence)
Intrasurgery TEE is recommended in patients undergoing surgery for IE	1 (level c evidence)
Diagnosis of IE in patients with persistent staphylococcus bacteremia without known cause	2a (level c evidence)
Diagnosis of IE in patients with in-hospital staphylococcus bacteremia	2b (level c evidence)

Modified from Bonow et al., ACC/AHA Practice guidelines, J Am Coll Cardiol 2006; 48:1–148.

initially negative examination may demonstrate vegetations 1–2 weeks later [8]. A known limitation of echocardiography is its inability to distinguish vegetations caused by infective endocarditis from aseptic ones that associate Libman–Sacks endocarditis and antiphospholipid syndrome [7].

Complications of NVE

TTE and, in particular, TEE have a pivotal role for the early detection and treatment of complications of infective endocarditis. The complications can be divided into valvular, para-valvular or others.

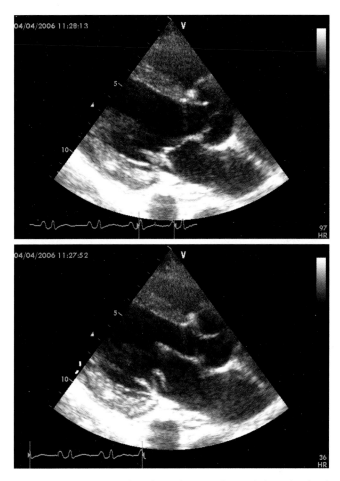

FIGURE 7.1.   TTE 2D imaging of vegetations of the mitral valve (posterior leaflet) during systole (*upper panel*) and diastole (*lower panel*) in parasternal long-axis view.

a) *Valvular complications*: The most important complication of NVE is valve regurgitation. This is caused by leaflet perforation, leaflet rupture, chordal rupture or complete valve destruction. Acute complications of significant

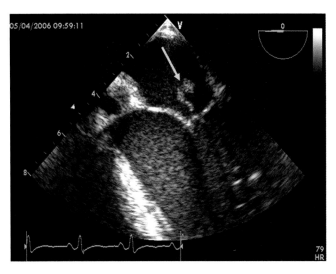

FIGURE 7.2. TOE showing a pedunculated vegetation of the mitral valve (see *arrow*) floating in the left atrial chamber.

magnitude may cause acute severe heart failure. Aortic cusp perforation and severe aortic valve regurgitation have been associated with poor prognosis unless urgent surgery is considered. Perforation of the mitral leaflets is less common (15% of endocarditis cases). In general, TTE seems to be more useful in detecting mitral than aortic perforation, with color Doppler allowing accurate detection of eccentric regurgitant jets that suggest leaflet perforation and that are distinguished from retrograde central orifice jets, commonly seen in native valves [7].

b) *Other complications*: The most important non-valvular complication is embolization. Embolic complications occur particularly with sizable vegetations (>10 mm). The risk of such large vegetations is three times that of small vegetations. Coronary artery embolization and abscess formation of the interventricular septum are much rarer complications. In view of the above, detailed

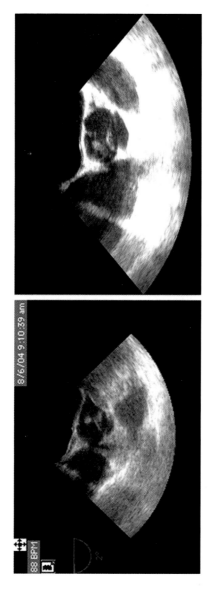

FIGURE 7.3. TEE showing multiple vegetations on the aortic valve. *Left panel*: diastolic frame, *right panel*: systolic frame.

TABLE 7.4. Echocardiographic surgical indications of infective endocarditis on native valves

Indications	Class
IF with valvular stenosis or regurgitation and heart failure.	1 (level b evidence)
IE with aortic and/or mitral regurgitation with hemodynamic consequences (increase of LV end-diastolic or atrial pressure, moderate- severe pulmonary hypertension).	1 (level b evidence)
IE caused by mycosis or microorganisms resistant to antibiotic therapy.	1 (level b evidence)
IE complicated by AV block, abscess of mitral/aortic annulus or fistula.	1 (level b evidence)
IE with recurrent embolic events and persistent vegetations despite antibiotic therapy.	2a (level c evidence)
IE with vegetation >10 mm (with or without embolism).	2b (level b evidence)

Modified from Bonow et al., ACC/AHA Practice guidelines, J Am Coll Cardiol 2006; 48:1–148.

echocardiographic examination has an invaluable role for establishing the indications for surgical management as stated in the ACC/AHA guidelines [2] (Table 7.4).

Prosthetic Valve Endocarditis (PVE)

PVE occurs on parts of a prosthetic valve or on a repaired native valve and accounts for up to 30% of all cases of infective endocarditis [9, 10]. PVE is either acquired peri-operatively (early PVE) or later after surgery (late PVE) [11, 12]. The first 12 months marks the early post-operative period during which the commonest causing organisms are S. *epidermidis and* S. *aureus* [13]. The diagnostic approach of PVE does not differ from that of NVE, however, the definitive diagnosis of PVE is often delayed because of the frequently delayed blood culture and echocardiographic confirming results compared to NVE [14]. Because of this the Duke criteria have a low sensitivity and cannot be applied [4]. PVE remains associated with bad prognosis, despite improvements in medical and surgical therapy [15].

Echocardiographic Approach

Diagnosis of PVE is established when typical clinical signs and symptoms are present and blood cultures are positive. Echocardiography further confirms the location of the valve infection by demonstrating vegetations on 2D images [16]. In the presence of mechanical prosthesis, a ring abscess may be the hallmark of infection which may lead to prosthesis dehiscence, para-valvular leak, extended infection to adjacent myocardial segments or even causing pericarditis. Mechanical valve stenosis is an uncommon evolution of endocarditis. Endocarditis of bioprostheses usually resembles that of native valves which includes valve stenosis and leaflet tear, perforation, flail or prolapse causing intraprosthetic regurgitation. Ring abscess and its complications are less frequent with bioprostheses. Septic embolization, metastatic abscesses, glomerulonephritis and mycotic aneurysms are potential but rare complications of both mechanical and biological valve endocarditis.

Although TTE is useful for diagnosing PVE, Figure 7.4, vegetations on prosthetic valves are more difficult to detect by TTE than those on native valves. The echogenicity of the sewing ring and supporting structures of mechanical and bioprosthetic valves prevent accurate identification of artificial valve infection and hence the serious indication for TEE for diagnosing PVE [7],. Figure 7.5. A recent survey [17] from 61 multinational centers has shown that TEE has been performed in 84% of suspected PVE compared to 68% of patients with NVE ($p<0.001$). This prevalence is justified by the fact that, while simple vegetations and new regurgitations

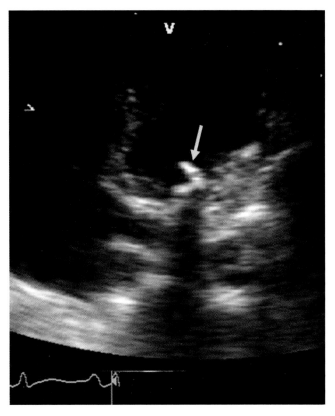

FIGURE 7.4.   TTE showing an IE vegetation (see *arrow*) of a mechanical mitral prosthesis (double hemi-disk), in apical four chamber view.

are much more commonly associated with NVE ring abscess is more frequently found in PVE compared to NVE (30% vs 12%, $p<0.001$). Accordingly, the sensitivity of TEE for diagnosing PVE is significantly higher than TTE [5, 18, 19], Figure 7.6. On the basis of these and other findings, the Task Force on Infective Endocarditis of the European Society of Cardiology has established a diagnostic algorithm for suspected PVE, where TEE has a crucial role, Figure 7.7. If

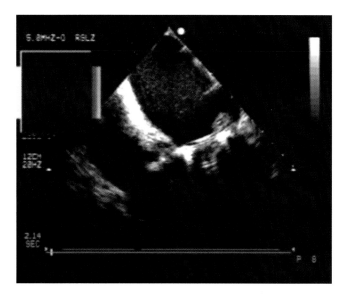

FIGURE 7.5.   TOE demonstrating PVE of the mitral valve.

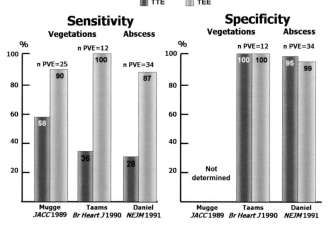

FIGURE 7.6.   Sensitivity and specificity of TTE and TOE for diagnosis of PVE.

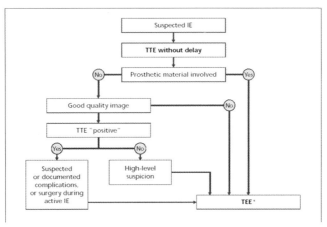

TTE "positive" indicates finding typical (i.e., fresh vegetation or abscess formation)

FIGURE 7.7.   Diagnostic algorithm for suspected PVE according to the ESC guidelines (modified from Ref. [12]).

TEE is negative and clinical suspicion is high, it should be repeated again after 48 h [20]

PVE-related Complications

1) Peri-annular complications. The known high incidence of peri-annular complications is due to the synthetic material of mechanical valves that does not allow microorganisms to grow, thus limiting its activity to the sewing ring [21–23]. Peri-annular complications frequently affect the mitral valve more than the aortic valve and may also cause AV block [24, 25]. On the other hand, bioprosthesis endocarditis begins on the surface of the leaflets and extends into its body resulting into tearing and perforation. Extension of infection to the para-valvular tissues usually carries a poor prognosis in the natural history of PVE. This includes endothelial erosion, peri-valvular abscess, pseudoaneurysms and intracardiac fistulae. TEE is the ideal echo technique for diagnosing peri-annular complications. In a retrospective analysis from 87 patients with anatomically proven PVE, TEE has shown a sensitivity of 90% for abscess and 100% for diagnosing pseudoaneurysms and fistulae [24].

2) Peri-valvular abscesses are not uncommon in PVE. The main diagnostic echocardiographic criteria are para-valvular cavity that changes its shape in the cardiac cycle with no blood flow inside, as well as valve rocking and para-prosthetic regurgitation, Figure 7.8. Abscesses should be differentiated from thrombus formation which are often associated with valve stenosis and abnormally mobile mass that is not necessarily associated with prosthetic valve regurgitation. Overall, definitive diagnosis of peri-valvular complications should be guided by the clinical history and blood cultures. While interrupted anticoagulation can result in thrombus formation prolonged fever and signs of septicemia may cause abscess formation.

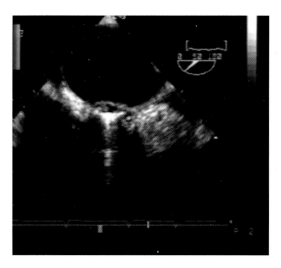

FIGURE 7.8.   Peri-valvular abscess of a prosthetic mitral valve.

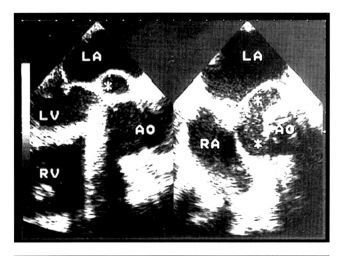

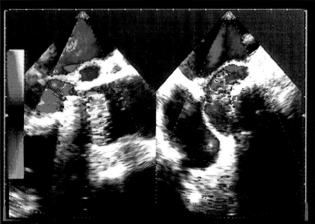

FIGURE 7.9.   ToE visualization of a pseudoaneurysm, *top panel* shows an echo-free peri-aortic cavity (see *asterisk*), *bottom panel* shows color Doppler of a flow communicating with aorta (AO). LA: left atrium, LV: left ventricle, RV: right ventricle (modified from Ref. [24]).

If ignored an abscess may expand to form a pseudoaneurysm which may subsequently perforate.

3) Para-valvular pseudoaneurysm is an echo-free cavity which is directly communicating with cardiac chambers as shown by color Doppler. A pulsatile echo-free para-valvular pouch with systolic expansion and diastolic emptying is a sensitive diagnostic criterion [24], Figure 7.9. Pseudoaneurysms are frequently located posteriorly, in the region between the base of the anterior mitral leaflet, the medial wall of the left atrium and the posterior aortic root. With changes in intracavity pressures aortic abscesses and pseudoaneurysms may rupture into the adjacent chambers causing intracavity fistulae. The echocardiographic features of a fistula is a narrow communication with continuous flow between two neighboring cavities, Figure 7.10. Fistulae may be single or multiple, commonly between the aorta and either the right or the left

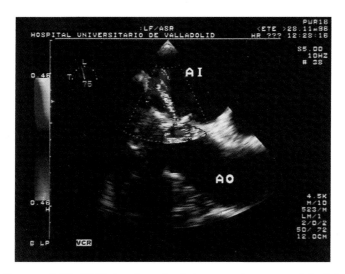

FIGURE 7.10. TEE showing a fistula between the aorta and the left atrium in a patient with a mechanical aortic prosthesis. AO: aorta, LA: left atrium (modified from Ref. [24]).

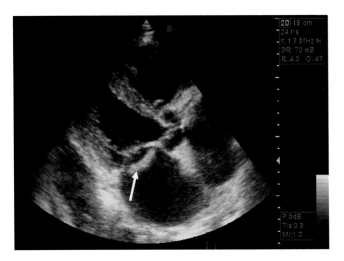

FIGURE 7.11. Partial detachment of a mitral prosthetic ring due to suture dehiscence. Note the separation between the mitral annulus and the prosthetic ring (*arrow*).

atrium [25]. Color Doppler identifies the site of communication and the potential cause and continuous wave Doppler confirms the exact timing of the communication flow [7].

4) Prosthesis dehiscence Another serious complication of PVE is prosthesis dehiscence which involves various degrees of valve detachment. A loose stitch is not uncommon but partial detachment, particularly in the presence of clinical and microbiological evidence for infection, is very suggestive of PVE, Figure 7.11. In this case, valve regurgitation is clearly seen on 2D echocardiographic imaging, and its quantification determines management plan [26].

PVE: Who Requires Surgery?

Although conventionally surgery is the best management option for PVE, guidelines based on prospective randomized trials are lacking. In a recent multicenter study of 104

TABLE 7.5. Echocardiographic surgical indications of Infective endocarditis on valvular prostheses (ESC guidelines)

Guidelines on prevention, diagnosis and treatment of infective endocarditis

Early PVE (<12 months after surgery)

Late PVE (>12 months after surgery complicated by:
- prosthesis dysfunction including peri-valvular leaks or obstruction, persistent positive blood cultures, abscess formation
- conductrion abnormalities
- large vegetations (>10 mm), particularly if staphylococci are the infecting agents.

Modified from Task Force of Infective Endocarditis of the ESC, Eur Heart J 2004; 25:267–276.

cases, Habib et al. concluded that (a) PVE not only carries a high risk for in-hospital mortality but also is associated with high long-term mortality; (b) early PVE, particularly caused by staphylococcal infection, development of complicated PVE or congestive heart failure are associated with bad outcome; (c) subgroups of patients could be identified for whom early surgery may result in better outcome, e.g., patients with staphylococcal and complicated PVE [27]. On these grounds, both ESC [12] (Table 7.5) and AHA/ACC guidelines [2] (Table 7.6) strongly recommend surgery for PVE.

Practical Indications

Echocardiography is the imaging investigation of choice for all cases with clinical suspicion of endocarditis, in addition to routine laboratory findings and microbiology. A negative TTE of good quality images may suggest an alternative diagnosis, particularly when the clinical grounds for the diagnosis are weak. With clear clinical or microbiological evidence TEE is imperative which should be repeated weekly if the first study was not conclusive.

TABLE 7.6. Echocardiographic surgical indications of infective endocarditis on valvular prostheses

Indications	Class
Heart failure, prosthetic detachment.	1 (level b evidence)
IE on valvular prosthesis (consult with surgeon), increase of trans-prosthetic gradient or regurgitation worsening.	1 (level c evidence)
Persistent bacteremia or recurrent embolism despite appropriate antibiotic therapy.	2a (level c evidence)
Cardiac surgery is not indicated in a first episode of prosthetic valve IE caused by a microorganism sensitive to antibiotic therapy.	3

Modified from Bonow et al., ACC/AHA Practice guidelines, J Am Coll Cardiol 2006; 48:1–148.

References

1. Durack DT, Lukes AS, Bright DK. New criteria for diagnosis of infective endocarditis: utilization of specific echocardiographic findings. Duke Endocarditis Service. Am J Med 1994; 96: 200–209.
2. Bonow RO, Carabello B, de Leon AC, ACC/AHA 2006 guidelines for the management of patients with valvular heart disease. Executive Summary. A report of the American College of Cardiology/American Heart Association Task Force on Practice Guidelines (Committee on Management of Patients With Valvular Heart Disease). J Am Coll Cardiol 2006; 48:1–148.
3. Jassal DS, Aminbakhsh A, Fang T. Diagnostic value of harmonic transthoracic echocardiography in native valve infective endocarditis: comparison with transesophageal echocardiography. Cardiovasc Ultrasound 2007; 5:20.
4. Sanfilippo AJ, Picard MH, Newell JB, Rosas E, Davidoff R, Thomas JD, Weyman AE. Echocardiographic assessment of patients with infectious endocarditis: prediction of risk for complications. J Am Coll Cardiol 1991; 18:1191–1199.

5. Mugge A, Daniel WG, Frank G. Echocardiography in infective endocarditis: reassessment of prognostic implications of vegetations size determined by transthoracic and the transesophageal approach. J Am Coll Cardiol 1989; 14:631–638.

6. Reynolds HR, Jagen MA, Tunick PA, Kronzon I. Sensitivity of transthoracic versus transesophageal echocardiography for detection of native valve vegetations in the modern era. J Am Soc Echocardiogr 2003; 16:67–70.

7. Evangelista A, Gonzalez-Alujas MT. Echocardiography in infective endocarditis. Heart 2004; 90:614–617.

8. Sochowski RA, Chan KL. Implications of negative results on a monoplane transesophageal echocardiographic study in patients with suspected infective endocarditis. J Am Coll Cardiol 1993; 21:216–221.

9. Edmunds LH, Jr., Clark RE, Cohn LH, Grunkemeier GL, Miller DC, Weisel RD. Guidelines for reporting morbidity and mortality after cardiac valvular operations: The American Association for Thoracic Surgery, Ad Hoc Liaison Committee for Standardizing Definitions of Prosthetic Heart Valve Morbidity. Ann Thorac Surg 1996; 932–935.

10. Vongpatanasin W, Hillis LD, Lange RA. Prosthetic heart valves. N Engl J Med 1996; 335:407–416.

11. Piper C, Korfer R, Horstkotte D. Prosthetic valve endocarditis. Heart 2001; 85:590–593.

12. Horstkotte D, Follath F, Gutschik E, Lengyel M, Oto A, Pavie A, Soler-Soler J, Thiene G, von Graevenitz A, Priori SG, Garcia MA, Blanc JJ, Budaj A, Cowie M, Dean V, Deckers J, Fernández Burgos E, Lekakis J, Lindahl B, Mazzotta G, Morais J, Oto A, Smiseth OA, Lekakis J, Vahanian A, Delahaye F, Parkhomenko A, Filipatos G, Aldershvile J, Vardas P. Guidelines on prevention, diagnosis and treatment of infective endocarditis. Eur Heart J 2004; 25:267–276.

13. Karchmer AW, Gibbons GW. Infections of prosthetic heart valve disease and vascular grafts. In: Bisno AL, Waldvogel FA, editors. Infections Associated with Indwelling Medical Devices. Washington: ASM Press, 1994; 213–249.

14. Habib G, Thuny F, Avierinos JF. Prosthetic valve endocarditis: current approach and therapeutic options. Prog Cardiovasc Dis 2008; 50:271–281.

15. Dajani AS, Taubert KA, Wilson W, Bolger AF, Bayer A, Ferrieri P, Gewitz MH, Shulman ST, Nouri S, Newburger JW,

Hutto C, Pallasch TJ, Gage TW, Levison ME, Peter G, Zuccaro G, Jr. Prevention of bacterial endocarditis: recommendations by AHA. Circulation 1997; 96:358–366.

16. Durack DT. Prevention of infective endocarditis, N Engl J Med 1995; 322:38–44.

17. Wang A, Athan E, Pappas PA, Fowler VG, Jr., Olaison L, Paré C, Almirante B, Muñoz P, Rizzi M, Naber C, Logar M, Tattevin P, Iarussi DL, Selton-Suty C, Jones SB, Casabé J, Morris A, Corey GR, Cabell CH. International Collaboration on Endocarditis-Prospective Cohort Study Investigators: Contemporary clinical profile and outcome of prosthetic valve endocarditis. JAMA 2007; 297:1354–1361.

18. Taams MA, Gussenhoven EJ, Bos E, de Jaegere P, Roelandt JR, Sutherland GR, Bom N. Enhanced morphological diagnosis in infective endocarditis by transoesophageal echocardiography. Br Heart J 1990; 63:109–113.

19. Daniel WG, Mügge A, Martin RP, Lindert O, Hausmann D, Nonnast-Daniel B, Laas J, Lichtlen PR. Improvement in the diagnosis of abscesses associated with endocarditis by transesophageal echocardiography. N Engl J Med 1991; 324: 795–800.

20. McFarland MM. Pathology of infective endocarditis. In: Kaye D, editor. Infective Endocarditis. New York: Raven Press, 1992; 57–83.

21. Zussa C, Galloni MR, Zattera GF, Pansini S, di Summa M, Poletti GA, Ottino G, Morea M. Endocarditis in patients with bioprostheses: pathology and clinical correlations. Int J Cardiol 1984; 6:719–735.

22. Calderwood SB, Swinski LA, Waternaux CM, Karchmer AW, Buckley MJ. Risk factors for the development of prosthetic valve endocarditis. Circulation 1985; 72:31–37.

23. Graupner C, Vilacosta I, SanRomán J, Ronderos R, Sarriá C, Fernández C, Mújica R, Sanz O, Sanmartín JV, Pinto AG. Periannular extension of infective endocarditis. J Am Col Cardiol 2002; 39:1204–1211.

24. San Román JA, Vilacosta I, Sarriá C, de la Fuente L, Sanz O, Vega JL, Ronderos R, González Pinto A, Jesús Rollán M, Graupner C, Batlle E, Lahulla F, Stoermann W, Portis M, Fernández-Avilés F. Clinical course, microbiologic profile, and diagnosis of periannular complications in prosthetic valve endocarditis. Am J Cardiol 1999; 83:1075–1079.

25. Chan KL. Early clinical course and long-term outcome of patients with infective endocarditis complicated by perivalvular abscess. Can Med Ass J 2002; 167:19–24.
26. Zabalgoitia M. Echocardiographic recognition and quantitation of prosthetic valve dysfunction. In: Otto C, editor, The Practice of Clinical Echocardiography, 3rd edn. Philadelphia: Saunders. 2007; 577–604.
27. Habib G, Tribouilloy C, Thuny F, Giorgi R, Brahim A, Amazouz M, Remadi JP, Nadji G, Casalta JP, Coviaux F, Avierinos JF, Lescure X, Riberi A, Weiller PJ, Metras D, Raoult D. Prosthetic valve endocarditis: who needs surgery? A multicentre study of 104 cases. Heart 2005; 91:954–959.

Index

A

Acquired aortic stenosis, 85–88
  calcific, 87
  rheumatic, 85–86
  senile or degenerative, 86–88
Active left ventricular cavity
      assessment, in aortic
      regurgitation, 129
Acute aortic regurgitation, 124
  management of, 140
Acute myocardial infarction,
      in ischemic mitral
      regurgitation, 31
Afterload reduction, in aortic
      regurgitation treatment,
      139–140
Annular calcification, mitral,
      28–29
Aortic dissection, 116
Aortic leaflet prolapse, 111–112
Aortic position
  valve obstruction in, 252–253
    pressure recovery, 252–253
Aortic regurgitation, 111–143, 229
  acute, 124
  aortic dissection, 116
  aortic leaflet prolapse, 111–112
  aortic valve infection
      (endocarditis), 112–113
  chest X-ray, 128

chronic, surgical intervention,
      140–143
clinical presentation, 125–126
dilatation of aortic root,
      113–116
echocardiography, 128–129
electrocardiography, 128
etiology, 111–118
investigations, 128–129
medical treatment, 137–139
  afterload reduction,
      139–140
  endocarditis prophylaxis,
      140
  root, 139
pathophysiology, 118–125
physical examination, 126–128
rheumatic disease of aortic
      valve, 111
severity, assessment, 129–137
  active left ventricular
      cavity, 129
  cardiac catheterization, 136
  coarse fluttering of anterior
      mitral leaflet, 129
  color flow jet diameter and
      area, 130–132
  color flow jet length,
      129–130
  continuity equation,
      134–139

Aortic regurgitation (*cont.*)
  continuous wave Doppler,
    132–134
  diastolic flow reversal, 134
  signs of, 127–128
  symptoms, 125–126
  syphilitic aortitis, 117–118
  treatment, 137–140
  ventricular septal defect,
    116–117
  See also Acute aortic
    regurgitation
Aortic stenosis, 73–111
  aortic gradient, determinants
    of, 74–75
  aortic valve area, 75
  aortic velocity, 75
  bicuspid aortic valves, 77
  breathlessness symptom,
    88–89
  chest pain symptom, 89–90
  clinical presentation, 88–93
  congenital aortic tubular
    stenosis, 80–81
  congenital cusp malformation,
    77
  coronary circulation in, 76–77
  echocardiography during,
    107–111
  etiology of, 77–88
  investigations, 93–94
    chest X-ray, 93
    echocardiography, 93–94
    electrocardiogram, 93
    transthoracic echocardiog-
      raphy, 93
  left ventricular response to, 76
  medical therapy, 102–103
  natural history, 100–102
  pathophysiology, 73–77
  physical examination, 91–93
  quadricuspid aortic valves, 77
  severity, assessment, 94–100
    cardiac catheterization, 100
    color flow Doppler, 98
    continuity equation, 96–99
    continuous wave Doppler,
      94–96
    leaflet separation extent, 94
    stress echocardiography,
      100
  subaortic stenosis, 81–85
  surgical treatment of, 103–107
    aortic valve replacement,
      104–107
    aortic valvuloplasty,
      103–104
    homografts, 105–107
    mechanical or bio-
      prosthetic valves,
      104–105
  symptoms, 88
  syncope symptom, 90–91
  treatment, 102–103
  See also Acquired aortic
    stenosis; Aortic
    regurgitation
Aortic valve disease, 73–143
  subvalvar aortic stenosis, 73
  supra-valvar aortic stenosis,
    74, 85
  See also Aortic stenosis
Aortic valve infection (endocardi-
    tis), 112–113
Aortic valve replacement, surgical
    treatment of, 104–107
Aortic valvuloplasty, surgical
    treatment of, 103–104
Arrythmia, 212–213, 216
Asymptomatic aortic stenosis
    with high-gradient, 228
Atrial fibrillation, 11
  in mitral valve disease, 28
Atrial septal defect, 162
Austin–Flint murmur, 127

B
Balloon valvuloplasty, 204
Bentall operation, 142

Bicuspid aortic valves, 77
Biological valves, 242–245
    advantage, 244
    disadvantage, 244
    Ross procedure, 244
Bioprosthetic valves, aortic
        stenosis, 104–105
Bjork–Shiley valve, 249, 260
Bleeding complication, in
        regurgitation, 260
Breathlessness symptom, in aortic
        stenosis, 88–89

C
Calcific aortic stenosis, 87
Carbomedics mitroflow, 243
Carcinoid disease, 160–161
Cardiac catheterization, 20
    in aortic regurgitation
        assessment, 136
    in aortic stenosis assessment,
        100
    dilated cardiomyopathy, 48–50
Cardiac magnetic resonance
        (CMR) technique
    in right ventricular size and
        function assessment,
        156
Cardiomyopathy, tricuspid
        regurgitation, 175
Carotid pulse examination, in
        aortic stenosis, 91
Carpentier–Edwards valve, 243
Chest pain symptom, in aortic
        stenosis, 89–90
Chest X-ray
    aortic stenosis, 93
    aortic regurgitation, 128
    rheumatic mitral stenosis,
        14–15
Chronic aortic regurgitation,
        surgical intervention,
        140–143
Closed mitral valvotomy, 25

Coarse fluttering of ante-
        rior mitral leaflet
        assessment, in aortic
        regurgitation, 129
Color flow Doppler
    in aortic stenosis assessment,
        98
    in pulmonary regurgitation
        assessment, 206
    in tricuspid regurgitation
        assessment, 182
Color flow jet length assessment,
        in aortic regurgitation,
        129–132
Congenital aortic tubular stenosis,
        80–81
Congenital cusp malformation,
        77–80
Congenital mitral stenosis, 4
Congenital tricuspid regurgita-
        tion, 171
Continuity equation, 20, 75
    in aortic regurgitation
        assessment, 134–139
    in aortic stenosis assessment,
        96–99
    dilated cardiomyopathy, 48
Continuous wave Doppler
    in aortic regurgitation
        assessment, 132–134
    in aortic stenosis assessment,
        94–97
    dilated cardiomyopathy, 45–47
    in pulmonary regurgitation
        assessment, 206
    in tricuspid regurgitation
        assessment, 184–187
Coronary artery disease in
        valvular heart disease
        patients, 232–233
Coronary circulation in aortic
        stenosis, 76–77
Coronary flow reserve in valvular
        heart disease patients,
        233–234

Corrigan's pulse, 127
Cyanosis, 214–216

D

Degree of valve calcification, mitral valve disease, 27–28
Dehiscence complication, in regurgitation, 260
Diastolic flow reversal assessment, in aortic regurgitation, 134
Dilatation of aortic root, 113–116
Dilated cardiomyopathy, 40–50
    mitral regurgitation severity, assessment of, 41–50
        cardiac catheterization, 48–50
        color flow area, 41–42
        continuity equation, 48
        continuous wave Doppler, 45–47
        large LV stroke volume, 41
        left atrial emptying volume, 48
        proximal isovelocity surface area (PISA), 42–43
        stress echocardiography, 48
        systolic flow reversal in pulmonary veins, 44–45
        three-dimensional color Doppler, 48
        vena contracta, 43–44
Disintegrating mitral bioprosthesis, 60–61
Dobutamine stress testing, in low-gradient aortic stenosis, 224–228
Duke criteria for infective endocarditis, 267–268
Durozier's sign, 127, 134
Dynamic subaortic stenosis, 83

E

Echocardiography
    aortic regurgitation, 128–129
    aortic stenosis, 93–94
    aortic valve replacement in elderly, 111
    during aortic valve surgery, 107–111
        intraoperative study, 108–109
        left ventricular dysfunction, 110–111
        post-operative assessment and follow-up, 109–110
        post-operative echo examination, 109
        pre-operative examination, 108
    for mitral valve disease
        assessing ventricular function, 27
        atrial fibrillation, 28
        degree of valve calcification, 27–28
        in patient selection for surgery, 27–28
    mitral valve prolapsed, 37
    percutaneous aortic valve replacement, 111
    of replacement valves, 245–250
        difficulties, 246
    surgical indications of IE on native valves, 274
    in valvular heart disease, 222
Elderly, aortic valve replacement in, 111
Electrocardiography
    aortic regurgitation, 128
    aortic stenosis, 93
    rheumatic mitral stenosis, 14–15
Embolic complications of native valve endocarditis, 272–274

Endocarditis, 265–284
   endocarditis prophylaxis, in
      aortic regurgitation
      treatment, 140
   See also Infective endocarditis;
      Native valve endocardi-
      tis (NVE); Prosthetic
      valve endocarditis
      (PVE)
Endocarditis, 62
   regurgitation, 258
   tricuspid, 173
Endomyocardial fibrosis
   causing mitral regurgitation,
      51–54
   tricuspid, 173

F
Fibrin strands/thrombi, 62–65
Flow convergence method, in
      mitral stenosis severity
      assessment, 16
Forward flow, replacement valves,
      248–249
Functional tricuspid stenosis,
      162–170
   atrial septal defect, 162
   clinical picture, 166
   investigations, 166–170
   localized pericardial effusion,
      162
   right atrial myxoma, 163
   right atrial secondaries,
      163–166

H
Homograft, 244
   in aortic stenosis, 105–107

I
Infective endocarditis
   diagnosis of, 266

Duke criteria for, 267–268
echocardiographic surgical
      indications of, 274
TTE indication for diagnosis
      of, 269–270
Inoue balloon valvuloplasty, 23
Interventional treatment, mitral
      valve disease, 22–27
   surgery, 25–27
      closed mitral valvotomy, 25
      mitral valve replacement,
         26–27
      open valvotomy, 25–26
      transesophageal echocardiog-
         raphy, 24
   valvuloplasty, 23–25
Intraoperative echocardiographic
      study, in aortic stenosis,
      108–109
Intraoperative transesophageal
      guidance, mitral
      regurgitation, 58–59
Ischemic mitral regurgitation,
      29–35
   acute myocardial infarction, 31
   clinical presentations, 31
   in a normal left ventricle, 32
   papillary muscle rupture, 32
   in ventricular dysfunction,
      32–33
Isolated mitral valve stenosis, 5

L
'Lack of contractile reserve', 225
Leaflet prolapse, tricuspid,
      174–175
Leaflet separation extent assess-
      ment, in aortic stenosis,
      94
Left atrial dilatation, 10–11
Left atrial emptying
      volume, dilated
      cardiomyopathy, 48

Left ventricular dysfunction, 13
  aortic stenosis with,
    223–228
  in aortic stenosis echocardiog-
    raphy, 110–111
Left ventricular response to aortic
    stenosis, 76
Low-gradient dysfunction, aortic
    stenosis with, 223–228
  dobutamine stress echo,
    224–228

M
Mechanical valves, aortic stenosis,
    104–105
Medtronic–Hall valve,
    249, 260
Mild hemolysis complication, in
    regurgitation, 260
Mitral position, valve obstruction
    in, 250–251
Mitral regurgitation, 29–64,
    230–232
  afterload, 35
  etiology of, 29–34
  follow-up after mitral valve
    surgery, 59–60
  intraoperative trans-
    esophageal guidance,
    58–59
  left atrium, 35
  management of, 55
  mitral valve repair, 57–58
  mitral valve replacement,
    56–57
  pathophysiology of, 34–36
  regurgitant orifice and jet, 34
  right heart, 35
  surgical intervention for,
    55–56
  uncommon causes of,
    51–54
    endomyocardial fibrosis,
    51–54

    ruptured chordae
      tendineae, 51
    See also Dilated cardiomy-
      opathy; Ischemic mitral
      regurgitation; Mitral
      valve prolapse
Mitral stenosis, 229–230
Mitral valve disease, 1–65
  echocardiography in patient
    selection for surgery,
    27–28
  follow-up, 22
  medical therapy, 22
  medical treatment of, 2
  mitral annular calcification,
    28–29
  mitral stenosis severity,
    assessment, 16–27
    cardiac catheterization, 20
    continuity equation, 20
    disease progress, 21
    flow convergence method,
    16
    mitral valve area, 16–22
    planimetry, 16
    pressure 1/2 time, 18
    transmitral pressure drop,
    18
    vena contracta, 16
  mitral stenosis, 4–7
    congenital mitral stenosis, 4
    isolated mitral valve
      stenosis, 5
    supra-valvar mitral
      stenosis, 5
  normal mitral valve anatomy
    and function, 2–4
  treatment, 22
    See also Interventional
      treatment
    See also Mitral regurgitation;
      Rheumatic mitral
      stenosis
Mitral valve prolapse, 35–40
  chocardiography, 37

clinical presentation, 36–37
investigations, 37–38
management, 39–41
    follow-up, 40
    medical therapy, 40
    natural history and
        complications, 38–39
    physical examination, 37
    specific gene defect for, 36
    symptoms, 36–37
    types, 36
        benign one, 36
        myxomatous leaflet
            disease, 36
Mitral valve repair, 57–58
    advantages, 59
    replacement versus, 59
Mitral valve replacement, 26–27,
        56–57
    mitral homograft, 56
    mitral valve prosthesis, 57
Mitral valve, 2–4
    anterior, 2
    components, 2
        annulus, 2
        chordate, 2
        leaflets, 2
        papillary muscles, 2
    normal, 2
Muscular subaortic stenosis, 83
Myxomatous mitral valve
        disease, 36

N
Native valve endocarditis (NVE),
        265
    complications of, 270–274
        embolic, 272–274
        valvular, 271–272
    diagnosis of, 266–270
Normal left ventricle, ischaemic
        mitral regurgitation in,
        32

O
Obstructed mitral prosthesis,
        61–62
Obstruction, valve, diagnosis,
        250–253
    aortic position, 252–253
    mitral position, 250–251
    tricuspid position, 253
Open valvotomy, 25–26

P
Pacemaker insertion, tricuspid,
        173–174
Pannus, regurgitation, 256–257
Papillary muscle rupture,
        in ischemic mitral
        regurgitation, 32
Paraprosthetic leaks, 254
Paraprosthetic regurgitation, 60
Para-valvular pseudoaneurysm,
        PVE-related, 281–282
Percutaneous aortic valve
        replacement, 111
Peri-annular complications,
        PVE-related, 278–279
Peri-valvular abscesses, PVE-
        related, 279–281
Planimetry, in mitral stenosis
        severity assessment, 16
Post-operative echo examination,
        in aortic stenosis, 109
    assessment, 109–111
    follow-up, 109–110
Pressure 1/2 time, in mitral steno-
        sis severity assessment,
        18
Primary failure, regurgitation, 256
Prosthesis dehiscence, PVE-
        related, 282
Prosthetic valve endocarditis
        (PVE), 266, 274–278
    echocardiographic approach,
        275–278
    practical indications, 283–284

Prosthetic valve endocarditis
(PVE) (*cont.*)
related complications, 278–282
para-valvular pseudoa-
neurysm, 281–282
peri-annular complications,
278–279
peri-valvular abscesses,
279–281
prosthesis dehiscence, 282
surgery, 282–283
Proximal isovelocity surface
area (PISA)/Proximal
isovelocity convergence
technique
dilated cardiomyopathy, 42–43
in tricuspid regurgitation
assessment, 182–184
Pseudoabscess, 259
Pulmonary autograft operation, in
aortic stenosis, 107
Pulmonary hypertension, 11–12
Pulmonary regurgitation,
205–218
arrythmia, 212–213
assessment, 206–209
color Doppler, 206
continuous wave Doppler,
206
complications of, 209–216
management, 216–218
restrictive right ventricular
disease, complications
of, 214
right ventricular dilatation,
209
right ventricular dysfunction,
209
right ventricular function,
assessment of, 213–216
Pulmonary stenosis, 196–205
clinical picture, 203–205
management, 203–205
severity, 200–203
subvalvar, 200–201

supravalvar, 201–203
valvular stenosis, 196–200
Pulmonary valve disease, 195–218
See also Pulmonary regurgitation; Pulmonary
stenosis

Q
Quadricuspid aortic valves, 77
Quinck's pulse, 127

R
Radiotherapy, tricuspid regurgitation, 175
Regurgitation, replacement
valves, 249–250
Bjork–Shiley valve, 249
complications, 255–261
bleeding, 260
dehiscence, 260
endocarditis, 258
mild hemolysis, 260
pannus, 256
primary failure, 256
thromboembolism, 257
thrombosis, 256
diagnosis, 253–255
Medtronic–Hall valve, 249
quantification, 255
regurgitant orifice and jet,
mitral regurgitation, 34
Replacement valves, 241–262
appearance, 246–248
assessment, 245–250
classification, 241–245
designs of, 243
forward flow, 248–249
history of, 242
mechanical valves, 241
obstruction, diagnosis of,
250–253
regurgitation, 249–250

stentless valves, 247
See also Biological valves
Residual tricuspid regurgitation, 190
Restrictive right ventricular disease
    complications of, 214–216
        arrhythmia, 216
        cyanosis, 214–216
        right heart failure, 216
Reversed septal movement, in tricuspid regurgitation assessment, 187
Rheumatic disease
    of aortic valve, 111
    rheumatic aortic stenosis, 85–86
    tricuspid, 171–173
Rheumatic mitral stenosis, 7–15
    atrial fibrillation complication, 11
    clinical presentation, 13–14
        physical examination, 13
        symptoms, 13
    complications of, 10–13
    investigations, 14–15
        chest X-ray and electrocardiogram, 14
    left atrial dilatation complication, 10–11
    left ventricular dysfunction, 13
    pathophysiology, 7
    pulmonary hypertension, 11–12
    right heart disease, 12
Rheumatic pulmonary stenosis, 199
Rheumatic valve disease, 1, 160
Right atrial myxoma, 163
Right atrial secondaries, 163–166
Right heart valve disease, 12, 155–191, 216
    regurgitation, diagnosis, 157–158
    tricuspid valve disease, 158

valve stenosis, diagnosis, 157–158
    ventricular response to, 155–156
    ventricular size and function, assessment, 156–157
    See also Tricuspid regurgitation; Tricuspid stenosis
Right ventricular dilatation, 209
Right ventricular dysfunction, 209
Right ventricular function, assessment, 213–216
Right ventricular pacing, 161
Root, aortic, treatment, 139
Ross procedure
    in aortic stenosis, 107
    in biological valves, 244
Ruptured chordae tendineae, causing mitral regurgitation, 51

S
Senile or degenerative aortic stenosis, 86–88
Simpson's rule, 98
Starr–Edwards valve in the mitral position, 63
Stentless valves, 247, 250
Stress echo in valvular heart disease, 221–236
    aortic stenosis with left ventricular dysfunction, 223–228
    aortic stenosis with low-gradient dysfunction, 223–228
    asymptomatic aortic stenosis with high-gradient, 228
    echocardiography applications in, 222
Stress echocardiography
    in aortic stenosis assessment, 100

Stress echocardiography (*cont.*)
    in coronary and valvular heart
        diseases, 235
    dilated cardiomyopathy, 48
Subaortic stenosis, 81–85
    dynamic, 83
    muscular, 83
Subvalvar aortic stenosis, 73
Subvalvar pulmonary stenosis,
    200–201
Supra-aortic stenosis, 85
Supra-valvar aortic stenosis, 74
Supra-valvar mitral stenosis, 5
Supravalvar pulmonary stenosis,
    201–203
Syncope symptom, in aortic
        stenosis, 90–91
Syphylitic aortitis, 117–118
Systolic flow reversal in
        pulmonary veins, 44–45

T
Three-dimensional color
        Doppler, dilated
        cardiomyopathy, 48
Thromboembolism, regurgitation,
    257
Thrombosis, regurgitation, 256
Transesophageal echocardio-
        graphy, mitral valve
        disease, 24
Transmitral pressure drop, in
        mitral stenosis severity
        assessment, 18
Transthoracic echocardiography
        (TTE), 266–283
    aortic stenosis, 93
    drawbacks, 275
    in infective endocarditis
        diagnosis, 269
    in NVE diagnosis, 266
Tricuspid position, valve
        obstruction in, 253

Tricuspid regurgitation, 12,
        171–191
    assessment of, 182–191
    cardiomyopathy, 175
    clinical picture, 177–182
    color flow Doppler in, 182
    congenital, 171
    continuous wave Doppler in,
        184–187
    endocarditis, 173
    endomyocardial fibrosis, 173
    etiology, 171–177
    functional, 171
    leaflet prolapse, 174–175
    medical treatment, 188–190
    pacemaker insertion, 173–174
    pathophysiology, 175–177
    proximal isovelocity conver-
        gence technique in,
        182–184
    radiotherapy, 175
    reversed septal movement in,
        187
    rheumatic disease, 171–173
    surgical procedures, 190–191
    treatment, 188
Tricuspid stenosis, 158–170
    carcinoid disease, 160
    etiology, 158–170
    rheumatic valve disease, 160
    right ventricular pacing, 161
    treatment, 170
        medical, 170
        surgical, 170
    See also Functional tricuspid
        stenosis

V
Valve prostheses, 232
Valve replacement complications,
    60–65
    disintegrating mitral biopros-
        thesis, 60–61
    endocarditis, 62

fibrin strands/thrombi, 62–65
obstructed mitral prosthesis,
        61–62
paraprosthetic regurgitation,
        60
Valve substitutes, *see* Replace-
        ment valves
Valvular complications of native
        valve endocarditis,
        271–272
Valvular heart disease
    coronary artery disease in
        patients with, 232–233
    coronary flow reserve in
        patients with, 233–234
    discordant symptoms, 229–230
    mitral regurgitation, 230–232
    mitral stenosis, 229–230
    stenosis severity, 229–230

stress echo in, 221–236
    See also Stress echo
stress echocardiography, 235
valve prostheses, 232
    See also Aortic regurgitation
Valvular stenosis, 196–200
Valvuloplasty, mitral valve
        disease, 23–25
Vena contracta
    dilated cardiomyopathy, 43–44
    in mitral stenosis severity
        assessment, 16
Ventricular dysfunction,
        ischaemic mitral
        regurgitation in, 32–33
Ventricular function assessment,
        for mitral valve disease,
        27
Ventricular septal defect, 116–117